CHRISTINE KACZMAR, D.C.

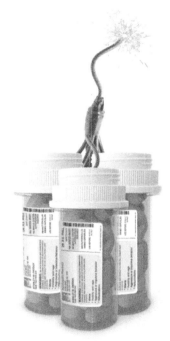

GUT CHECK

How The Broken Medical Model
Is Creating More Sickness
And Why Timeless Healing Principles Are Needed Now

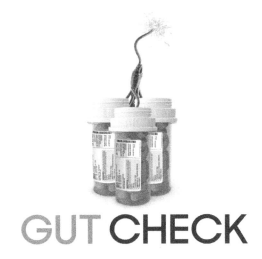

GUT CHECK

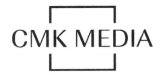

CMK MEDIA

Published by CMK Media Group, Shelby Township, Michigan (586) 685-2222

CMK Media books may be purchased for educational, business, or sales promotional use. For information, please email hello@thedigestiondoctor.com or contact Patti at 586-685-2222

First Edition, Printed in USA

Cover Design: Penny O'Brien, Enrique Gomez, Christine Kaczmar
Layout Design: Laurie Metanchuk, David Santilli
ISBN 978-1-7327722-0-5

Acknowledgments:

To my Mom: Thank you for contributing to my most treasured gift... freedom. Growing up, you gave me the autonomy I needed which made all of the difference. I am forever grateful for the space you gave me to become who I am. You never interfered, confined, or smothered me. Thank you for tirelessly believing in me even when you wanted to strangle me. I hope this book makes you proud. I love you, Mom.

To Laurie, Scotty, and Marky: Look how we turned out, eh? Thank you for accompanying me on this ride through a lens only we share. It's time for a croquet marathon. Uncle Dick calls blue.

To Sue: Thank you for being the calming force in my professional life. Your addition to the team was a true turning point and your presence always gives me comfort. Thank you for understanding who I am and recognizing my rough edges are only temporary. You are an inspiration in ways you cannot imagine.

To Lisa: Thank you for being the bright light in my life. Our friendship means the world to me. Wiley Coyotes Forever!

To Patty: You are my soul sister. I cannot thank you enough for your friendship, counsel, and support. Corn nuts and road trips ASAP. Ok?

To Dr. Loomis: Your extensive knowledge in enzyme nutrition shifted my life in ways in which I could never thank you enough. I have limitless gratitude for your life's work and devotion to teaching. Words cannot express how deeply I value you...

To every patient who gave me the chance to make a difference in your life. Thank you for the opportunity. I am so fortunate to have the very best patients in the world. This book is for you. Finally, to every Rebel carrying a chip on their shoulder... keep seeking the truth with a defiant spirit and relentless pursuit. You are the giants who stand tall when it isn't popular or even safe. This book is absolutely for you.

Table of Contents

A note from Dr. Christine

Before you get cracking into this book, I want to explain one thing. I thoroughly enjoy quotes. I love to pick up a book, flip to a random page and dive in. If you have any similar tendencies, you will especially appreciate what I have done here. Throughout the GUT-Check book, I have purpose-fully gone heavy-handed on the quotes and quick tips. My point in doing this is to highlight the very important aspects to gut health and digestion. Once you finish the book, come back to it when you have even a few moments and revisit the call-out text and "GUT-Check Goodies"

As always...

Love Yourself Healthy,

CHAPTER 1: 'The Loomis Effect'

"You either take charge and create your future, or you let someone else do it. The choice is yours." — James Mapes

The year was 2007. Chicago, Illinois. The hotel was nothing ultra fancy, but the inside of the seminar room looked sharp. I took my place at the front of the room. I liked the comfort of the chair. It was black, cushy, and it spun around. I took a quick look and liked what I saw. The atmosphere felt comfortable. Academic learning vibes were in the air. Ah yes, learning, something I have been addicted to since I was a young girl. Today was no different. Perhaps the only distinction about this day was my first impression. It stood out. Why? As a person who constantly bird-dogs new information and educational advantages, this conference had more riding on it than I could have ever predicted.

I was attending my first Loomis Institute educational seminar entitled "Seminar One: Loomis Digestive Health Specialist." My inner thoughts were those of a composed, *'Let's see what you've got, Dr. Loomis.'* Since I had heard his name mentioned quite a few times, and had seen his articles in numerous publications, I felt eager anticipation to see what he had to say. I was about to witness if he indeed stood up to his esteemed reputation and outstanding recommendations from my colleagues.

My recollection of the exact words he opened the conference with are scant. What I do remember is that within the early moments of his initial remarks, he struck a deep chord in me. He articulated the connection between structure and function. It rang true. It made me move forward in my leather chair and listen closer. I leaned in, way in. Was it possible that this was a game-changing seminar for my professional career? Was it possible that this man I had heard about for the last seven years was going to be of great impact and influence in my life? These thoughts flashed through my mind like little gold sparks of creative promise. I knew my attendance there was anything but a coincidence.

What further made this an interesting situation was the timing. You see, I had literally just quit my job as an associate chiropractic doctor. Understand something, I am not employable. Let me take you back a few years and explain what I mean.

When I first graduated chiropractic school, I moved to New England. Naturally, I worked for another doc. That is what newly-minted graduates do. They team up with senior doctors in the field to get experience and hopefully the beginnings of a patient base. In my case, the working-for-another-person adventure only lasted for a few months before I knew I had to invoke an exit strategy.

The final straw or, ahem, "shred" was when the senior doctor bought a paper shredder. For 40-minutes, he fancifully sat there enjoying his new toy. Once he was done, he nonchalantly directed me to clean up his paper-fragment nightmare. There were thousands of white remnants strewn about the burgundy carpet. *'Excuse me,'* I thought. *'Is this guy for real?'* Without incident, I kept my violated thoughts to myself. I retrieved the vacuum and sucked his shredder shrapnel into the Hoover.

'I need to get out of here. I need to really, really, really get out of this place. How will I do it? How will I finance it? I am less than 6 months out of chiropractic school, how will I swing this? I just will,' I thought. *'I just will.'* I went home for lunch and began charting my course to employment freedom.

Within 40 days of the puny paper caper, I opened my first practice. Soon, I owned and operated two locations. It was a grind because I felt incomplete. Despite the independence and joy working for yourself provides, I honestly missed my home state. I craved the diversity and culture that Michigan offered. With a heavy heart, I made the decision to return home. I secured a fancy agency to help me sell my practices. Shortly before closing the deal, the potential buyer's financing collapsed. The impending move date, however, was firm. This was tragic. Without this buyer in place, I had to scramble to find a new buyer. In the end, I basically walked away with nothing, because the only doc I remotely liked in the neighboring area was fresh out of school — and broke.

I moved back to Michigan knowing I would temporarily have to associate for another doc again. It helped that the office I would be running was one of five that this doctor owned. The geography of his practices were very spread out. This particularly appealed to me because I wanted the most autonomy as humanly possible. For the most part, I had that, but it wasn't enough. This doctor had his eye on the stats and the stats alone. He didn't have a lot to say or a lot to discuss. My responsibilities were to run his practice and call him every night with the numbers.

The numbers included various statistics: patient visits, new-patient conversions, and the number of no-shows. As the end of each working night approached, a feeling of dread washed over me. I would need to call this doctor with the stats. Now this may not seem like such a pain in the ass, but it was. He would grill me if a new consult did not convert after receiving their free spinal exam from the previous night's telemarketing call. If the people who came in for their free exam decided against a chiropractic care schedule, I was blamed.

In the short four months I ran his practice, I more than tripled Dr. X's bottom line. My educational style and patient care provided a consistent force that was reflected in the numbers, but it was never enough for Dr. X. Finally, on the morning of a weekly staff meeting, on the day after our busiest week ever, he was again, dissatisfied. In fact, he was critical, so critical that I felt the blood rushing to my head. I was disgusted. There I was, burdened with another session of statistical torture. Don't get me wrong, Dr. X was highly revered, but his words were imbued with emotional disconnect. People are so much more than mere numbers. Even so, Dr. X was short on compliments and heavy on disappointment. Nothing would ever be enough for him. I had heard enough. Before another moment passed, I rose up from my chair and said, "I can't do this. I can no longer work for you." Away I went. Dr. X tried to calm me down, but his efforts were too late. My decision had been made. I could take no more. I vowed to never be employed again. I needed to be my own boss.

Initially, I felt overwhelmed with power. I remember the surging presence of adrenaline in my body. But, this silent, celebratory cheer was short-lived. With my reactive and rebellious decision, I put myself at great risk. I did not financially plan for this. I was not prepared to live without a paycheck. Who really is? The very next morning, my spirited workplace anarchy morphed into debilitating panic. Did I just make the biggest mistake of my career? It was November. Holiday time was in full swing. The snowflakes were flying and Bing Crosby was singing on the radio. Shoppers were spending their hard-earned dollars on Christmas presents. Who in their right mind opens up a new business during holiday time? Apparently, I do.

I swallowed my pride and I got to work. I had no choice. For three months, it was an uphill climb, but slowly I began to build my new practice, the way I've always wanted to, with not just chiropractic but incorporating a functional medicine approach, as well.

Despite the terrible timing of building a brand-new practice and facing economic hardship, I decided to fly out to Chicago to attend my first digestive-health conference, the very conference I opened the chapter with here, Dr. Loomis' event. It was a risky decision, but one I instinctively made.

You know how fate works its magic? Well, after the 3-days with the incredible Dr. Loomis concluded, I arrived at the airport to find that all flights to Detroit were canceled. To this day, I never found out why. There was no storm. There was no explanation.

I considered renting a car to make the 6-hour overnight commute, but instead, ruled in favor of my "purposeful" circumstance. There must be a reason for this, I thought. I actively worked on suppressing my feelings of incredible anxiety. I was anxious because I had secured a very important speaking gig at a local hospital for the next day. As a functional-medicine doc, there are not many opportunities to get in front of medical doctors and their staff. It took so long to get past the gatekeepers to schedule this event, and to miss this shot was quite stressful.

I weighed my options, and asked to be booked on a flight for the next morning. Now, here comes the silver lining. That night and into the next day, I embarked on a special study session. I used this extra time to gain traction on what I learned from the digestive conference. I meticulously reviewed everything. I knew the information made sense. Now, I would need to implement what I had learned. There was no time to lose. More importantly, I needed to see if the application of all I learned actually worked. Would the plant enzymes I studied about make a positive change in my patients' digestive health? I began to create a system of just how I would introduce this new testing method into my practice. While at the gate inside O'Hare, I devised my first marketing materials. I constructed everything necessary to hit the ground running. In the end, it is because of this flight delay that my digestive practice was established.

Now, you may be reading this and perhaps not connecting how a chiropractic doctor — a doctor of the spine and nervous system, — would have any desire to expand into the digestive space. Here is what you may not know. When I entered chiropractic school, I was in the worst shape of my life. I weighed north of 230 pounds. I ate all the cookies I wanted, and I seldom exercised. Strange as it sounds, I was always a successful athlete throughout my school years. Sports came naturally to me. Once I left collegiate softball and tennis behind, I left regular and structured exercise behind as well.

During my prerequisite and advanced organic chemistry courses, and while amongst a community of healthier-looking people, I began to understand how wretched my health truly was. I knew changes must be made. For the six to seven years prior to chiropractic school, I had become obese. I worked 60+ hour weeks in Michigan's largest drug store, Perry Drugs. Ironic, eh? Because of this ruthless schedule, it was difficult for me to prioritize my life. I was a slave to my schedule and I never exercised. Even if I did exercise, I still ate the Standard American Diet, a sad diet to be sure. In my midwestern household, we ate traditional foods that consisted of the packaged and processed variety. Fresh salads were seldom, if ever, at the supper table. In fact, I did not discover romaine lettuce, avocados, kombucha, etc., until I was 25 years old.

As I entered university to become a doctor, it was obvious that I looked different than the others. I was slightly older, and massively heavier than they were. Quite simply, I hardly knew anything about health. My typical habit was to walk to the local Blimpie sandwich shop and get their biggest turkey provolone sub with a two liter of Coke and a bag of chips. I would make the short trek home, my only exercise, and dive in. My favorite thing was to drink half of the 2-liter of pop, polish off the entire sandwich and most of the crunchy potato chips while watching *Melrose Place*.

Growing up in Michigan, I was accustomed to slurping down glasses of milk for "strong bone health." **Wrong**. I believed low-fat and high-carbohydrate diets were okay because this is what I heard someone say on television. **Wrong**. I thought taking cold and flu medicine and other prescription drugs were harmless and safe because I once worked for a pharmacy. Clearly everything they sell is safe. **Wrong**. I thought big pharmaceutical companies were honorable and had our best interests at heart. **Mega wrong**.

I knew nothing.

Every day, the more I learned about my body and all of its magnificence, the more angry, albeit elated, I became. I was angry because I felt so ignorant. Why in the world had I not learned any of this? I felt elated because I was now empowered. I was disentangling 25 years of lies. It was a lot to unwind. I was about to learn what health *really* was, and flip the script on a quarter-century's worth of false beliefs.

It has been said that we are the average of the five people with whom we spend the most time. Because of this truth, I transformed.

During my time at the university, I began to extensively learn about the body, diet, digestion, neurology, pathology, etc. I was amazed.

I began to see things differently. I began to move. In the fall of 1996, I bought a piece of workout equipment from my Mom's favorite channel, QVC. I ordered this funky little cross-country skiing gizmo. It was a big, black and red concave apparatus made of tough plastic. It had 2 rectangles to place your feet on, and two poles, one for each hand. I placed it in the spare bedroom and began my trans-formation. At first, I was demolished after 5 minutes. I decided to impose a rule, something small to create big-little victories. Before I was allowed to quit exercising, I would first have to listen to two songs of either Everything But The Girl or Sarah McLachlan.

It worked. I formed a routine. I began to take control, and it felt sensational. I remember moments in the beginning, when I would complete my workout after listening to an entire CD, and then collapse onto the beige-carpeted floor of my duplex rental and stare at the ceiling. As I struggled to catch my breath, I wondered what my life would be like when I got out of there. What would my life be like when I got even healthier, when I would make a meaningful contribution to the world?

After four to six weeks of my new exercise routine, I had a visit from my brother and his wife. I opened the door and I will never forget the reaction. My brother's wife said, "Chrissy, you are looking so good! You are losing weight!" I was delighted. This was my first confirmation that anything I was doing was making a difference. It perked me up and kept me going. The chiropractic education had expanded my mind in a way I had never known.

Oddly, after shedding 44 pounds and feeling like a new woman, something strange happened. I began noticing severe abdominal discomfort. I was eating the best I had ever eaten, exercising like a beast, yet there I was, doubled over in P.N.S. (peripheral nervous system) class. As the doctor lectured about afferent and efferent fibers, I sat crumpled up at my desk with my arms tightly wrapped around my belly. I was in pain. Why? I had just eaten a robust and healthy salad with my pals for our short lunch break. I was regularly engaging in trail running and various exercises. I had dropped a lot of weight, so none of these pains made any sense. Even when I was so much heavier, I had never experienced this kind of agony. Why was this sharp abdominal cramping becoming a more-frequent occurrence?

It wasn't until I discovered Dr. Paul Goldberg, affectionately referred to as "Small Paul," that my health and education took a meaningful detour. Dr. Goldberg lectured about diet, nutrition, vegetarianism, and the benefits of water-only fasting. I was enchanted. In fact, I was so eager about his teachings, that I made an appointment to see him during one of the short breaks between classes. I had to figure out what I was doing wrong because the belly cramping was crimping my style. I made the decision that I would do something drastic. I would embark on a water-only fast, guided by Small Paul, himself.

I knew I had to do it. I scrambled to get the money for the testing together, and my first water-only fast was under way. I felt confident that seeing Dr. Goldberg would provide an answer to why I was having severe abdominal pains. I water-only fasted for eight days. During this fast, my follow-up visits with Dr. Goldberg were every two to three days. On these visits, he would test a sample of my urine, take my pulse, inspect my tongue, look closely into my eyes, and ask me a few questions. On the eighth day, he felt it was sufficient time to end my fast. I had lost 11 pounds in this process, an added bonus, but certainly not the reason I conducted the fast. What was incredibly striking during the fast, and currently remains to be remarkable as I regularly water-only fast each year, is the way the tongue clears. When I say clears, I am referring to the return of a bright red and healthy tongue. Our tongues are superior indicators of our health. As for the results of my eight-day fast, suffice it to say, the severe and stabbing abdominal pain I suffered was gone. It never again returned. I knew that although I would graduate as a Doctor of Chiropractic, there was high value in what had just transpired. Should I ever require it in future practice, the digestive system would certainly have to be a part of my playbook. Of course, I will talk more about this later, but working with Dr. Goldberg was a massive and pivotal influence in not only my health but my business.

When I graduated chiropractic school in December 1999, I was one of the few people who left thinner and fitter than when I first entered. It is not hard to understand why someone would leave heavier than when they entered. The intensity of the curriculum and the time commitment to clinical requirements left a lot of room for convenient choices such as fast food, yummy candy, and comforting treats. For me, I completely revolutionized my life. I was ready. Bring on the world! I was a fresh new graduate with high goals, transformational health information, and plenty of energy. Let's go!

Now, back to being stuck at the Chicago airport. Within three days of returning home, my new marketing message was complete. Off I went, distributing my informational flyers. After a day or two, I had my first bite. An 83-year old man, Zack, was the first to contact my office. He was dealing with horrible and chronic diarrhea. I will never forget his comment to me when we met. He said I was his "last hope." This made my mission quite real. I could see the pain and frustration in his eyes. Even though I had very little training of the new system, I knew I had to help this man. I gathered the information from one of the urinary test kits I pre-ordered from the Chicago concourse. I gave Zack the instructions and sent him on his way. Within 48 hours, his results returned from the lab. 'Here it goes,' I thought. I gave him three product formulas based off of his digestive test results. His first checkup, post-product disbursement, was three days later. When he returned, Zack looked notably different. He was smiling, and believe it or not, he looked younger and more at ease. I was astonished, to be quite honest. Could it be that this enzyme nutrition stuff was for real? Keep in mind, this was the first patient I was using these products on, and it seemed to work fantastically. The best part of this story is that with each subsequent follow-up, Zack improved.

And so it went, I incorporated these methods on hundreds of patients with similar results: drastic improvements. As you can imagine, it didn't take long before I was convinced. The rest, as they say, is history.

I want to make an important point. You see, previous to working with enzyme nutritional therapies, I used to test for food allergies and sensitivities. This protocol didn't work. Despite the fact that patients would remove offending foods from their diets, their issues persisted. If testing the blood for food allergies and removing the food sensitivities from diets didn't accomplish improvements, then this testing structure had to be tossed out. And toss it out I did.

I think it would be incredibly refreshing for doctors — or any professional — to admit when something is not working. If this were a more-common practice, wouldn't that be fantastic? Ego plays a major role here. It just does. It is really too bad, because this arrogance is such a deterrent to healing. Healing is something that is rooted in authenticity and kindness. It is quite impactful to also consider the role hope plays in healing and recovery. But, in order to have this conversation, it is also paramount to discuss fear. You see, I can say with certainty that the medical profession has masterfully created disruption through fear-based medicine. People think they require a lot of potions, lotions, and pills in order to achieve true health.

When it comes to working with your medical professional, here are four questions I have for you:

1. Do you think your body is a brilliant machine that knows how to heal itself?

2. Do you feel your doctor truly listens to you with an open mind or do they seem authoritative?

3. Are you concerned that little discussion is given toward alternative solutions and that people are taking more prescription medications than ever?

4. Does your doctor ever discuss natural options with you before prescribing medications?

I hope your answer to question 1 is a resounding, 'Heck yeah!' If not, perhaps your mind will change once you've finished this book.

One of the things that is very apparent is that confusion exists. Whom do you believe? What diet does one follow? How can you determine which method is right for you? I completely understand this complicated inner dialogue. It makes perfect sense to me why so many people are frustrated and confused. Look, if being healthy were easy, everyone would be healthy. Similarly, how do you know that the doctor you are seeing will provide results? How do you know they can help you? How do you know what their track record is? Well, you don't. You have to, for a lack of a better word, go with your gut. Your gut makes a lot of decisions. If your instincts are not feeling it, you are probably right. If you have an inkling about something, dig deeper. Listen to your inner gut. Now is the time for a collective "gut check." Even though I was not aware of this with my upbringing, and despite learning it well into my 20s, if more people just contemplated and then embraced these timeless healing principles, lives would be saved. Here are three, timeless, healing principles that will forever remain true.

Timeless Healing Principles:

1.   The body knows how to heal itself.
2.   The body is constantly trying to stay in homeostasis.
3.   The body's primary defense system, known as the immune system, lives in the gut.

We have heard sayings such as: "Look well to the gut for the cause of disease" or "You are only as healthy as your digestive system," and so on. There is a reason these phrases have stood the test of time. They are true. In fact, your gut has its very own electrical panel. In other words, it has its own nervous system. This complex circuitry is known as the **enteric nervous system**. This brilliant wiring can make decisions independent of the brain. It can execute commands on a whim, and it does so every single second of the day. It's truly amazing! Your digestive system is a powerhouse. This book is all about making a "gut-check" toward better health, clearer choices, and healthier digestion.

Finally, it is never too late to change your perspective. I hope your mind is open to witnessing how you are blatantly being lied to, how you are boldly marketed to, how you must pay attention to the very best doctor, your body's inner doctor.

I am thankful for all of the lessons I have learned along the way, especially what I am calling "The Loomis Effect." This man has impacted my life more than he will ever know. In my personal experience, if I continued down the road without course correcting, my health would have significantly suffered. If I had not changed my habits, opened my mind, pursued learning something new — even when the timing wasn't perfect — who knows where I would be in my life or career right now. My hope is within these pages, you experience your own internal "gut-check." As an additional bonus from what you discover here, perhaps another Rebel is born.

CHAPTER 2: THE BROKEN MEDICAL MODEL

 "Doctors pour in drugs about which they know little to treat diseases of which they know less in human beings of which they know nothing." — Voltaire

Let's talk about medical ego in a modern era. Not only has ego complicated the healing process, but it has also damaged and killed thousands of people. Allow me to explain. I have a mission, a fierce mission. I boldly proclaim to you that my mission is to *save* 5 million lives from the broken medical model.

If you are still reading, and not put-off by such a lofty and perhaps downright arrogant assertion, hang with me for a moment. I get it.

America's first responders, emergency room trauma teams, specialty surgeons — they're second to none. Emergencies, crisis care, trauma... we need these doctors! I want to openly state my appreciation for the amazing artistry our country's physicians and nurses deploy each and every day. Whether it is surgically repairing a fractured spine, meshing a blown aorta, or striking other ways doctors save lives, I truly admire and respect these heroic and daily miracles. These doctors possess sensational and staggering levels of moxie, skill and talent. However, I am not talking about this kind of model or even these types of doctors.

No, my disgust lies elsewhere. It is positioned squarely at the traditional medical or allopathic model. I call it the "broken medical model."

Throughout this chapter, I have outlined four specific ways in which the traditional medical model is broken. I refer to them as "healing violations." They are violations because until the medical model radically changes, patients will continue to suffer and die.

Ego gets in the way because the current medical model, the broken medical model, has not *forgotten* but *chosen* to eliminate centuries of healthful healing practices in favor of greed. Today, chemists put on an embroidered, crisp, white, lab coat and go about tampering with Mother Nature in the name of science.

HEALING VIOLATION #1
Ego: The Body Is Ignorant

> **"Despite the tendency of doctors to call modern medicine an "inexact science," it is more accurate to say there is practically no science in modern medicine at all. Almost everything doctors do is based on a conjecture, a guess, a clinical impression, a whim, a hope, a wish, an opinion, or a belief."[1]** – Robert Mendehlson, M.D.

Give me a break. The audacity to think their creations are better suited for a human's healing consumption, rather than nature's pharmacy, is infuriating.

Big Pharma knows the truth. They have made their commitment, and it's not to safety, efficacy or results. In addition, too many medical professionals have chosen coin over common sense.

The broken medical model ignores Timeless Healing Principle #1: The body knows how to heal itself. Instead, their model is based on the idea that illness is treated from the outside, by some external force. All too often, this treatment involves the use of prescription medications.

> **"Medicine can support your body through an emergency, surgery can be necessary in certain circumstances, but it is only your own body that has the ability to heal."**[2] – Hiromi Shinya, M.D.

Prescription medications are not nutrients, nor do they nourish the body. Since only nutrition normalizes function, there is a significant disconnect, here. You cannot take something external, or in essence *foreign* to the body, like prescription drugs, and expect them to natively nourish the body like food does.

Let me say it again. Nutrition normalizes function. The best part about this is that human physiology is not going to change anytime soon. You can bank on the fact that food is what heals, especially if food is consumed in proper proportions and digested well. Food is the *real* medicine. There is not a doctor on the planet who can accurately predict how the non-nourishing ingredients found in a big pharmaceutical company's tablets or capsules will work inside each person's physiology. Not. One. Doctor. Can. Predict. This.

Instead, when doctors discuss function, they should extensively converse about deviations from the body's normal state. Where are the disruptions or dysregulations?

GUT-Check Goody

Attitude Problem? Take This Drug

"For most people, a gradual dysregulation in immune function — an impairment of the immune system's physiological regulating mechanism — is the norm. Unfortunately, the conventional medical community rarely recognizes the dysregulation. This is a significant problem in medicine today: if you don't suffer from a diagnosable disease for which a doctor can prescribe drugs, then the attitude of the medical profession is that there isn't anything wrong with you."[3] - Donald Yance

In the broken medical model's paradigm, the body is treated as *incapable* of healing itself. Their cavalier attitude is that the body needs pharmaceuticals, flu shots, vaccines and medications.

Sadly, it is inside these Big Pharma boardrooms, replete with shiny mahogany tabletops and copious 60-something year-old white men that the fate of many unsuspecting Americans begins. Within this sterile space, the next toxic prescription medication is devised, engineered and marketed. The more profitable the drug, regardless of patient safety, the better. The name of the game here is greed. The race to a patent is on. If they can patent their creations, this secures even more moolah.

To further insulate Big Pharma's protection, political influence is essential. Did you know that of all existing industries, pharmaceutical companies outspend all of them? That's right. Nobody drops more dollar bills to manipulate members of Congress like Big Pharma does.

> **"When buying and selling are controlled by legislation, the first thing to be bought and sold are legislators."** – P.J. O'Rourke, American Political Satirist

The fat wallets at Merck, Pfizer, Novartis, etc., keep banging out meds, while stuffing their pockets full of profits. This reality doesn't appear to be changing anytime soon.

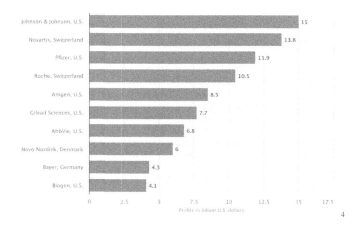

The most despicable part? Big Pharma is guilty of spending more money on marketing their poisons than on their safety and research. It is precisely this kind of advertising budget that brainwashes the masses, and bludgeons authentic methods for healing.

With Big Pharma's immense power came unchecked ego. Their sales recruitment didn't stop with medical doctors, it went well beyond that and straight to Washington, D.C.

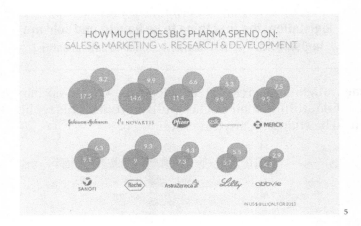

According to Gina Chon, who wrote a piece in *The New York Times* on Big Pharma spending, "Drug makers have been getting their $2.3 billion worth in Washington. That is how much they have spent lobbying Congress over the last decade. It may help explain why no legislative proposal to rein in rising prescription prices has gone anywhere.

All the while, the pharmaceutical industry has been spreading dollars around the nation's capital. Drug makers doled out $240 million for lobbying purposes last year, according to the Center for Responsive Politics, making it the biggest spender. The insurance industry was second, at $157 million."[6]

In Washington, money clearly controls and highly influences.
Can you see how problematic this is? They blatantly place profits ahead of results and safety. They will spin their twisted little tales

of "science" and make intelligent people think they need their latest compromising cocktail.

Pharmaceutical companies spend far more than any other industry to influence politicians. Drug makers have poured close to $2.5 billion into lobbying and funding members of Congress over the past decade.

The medical doctor's curriculum is dictated by Big Pharma. Did you know Big Pharma spends more money lobbying Congress than Big Oil?

At the time of this publication, nine out of 10 members of the U.S. House of Representatives and all but three of the 100 U.S. senators have taken campaign contributions from pharmaceutical companies, seeking to affect legislation on everything from the cost of drugs to how new medicines are approved.

Simply put, Big Pharma's stacks of cash help create new governing beliefs. People witness thousands of advertisements with brilliant marketing techniques, jingles, and delivery systems. How do you spell relief? What is the purple pill? What is the pink stuff? What is the blue triangular pill for men? Ask anyone over 45 years old, and chances are solid that they can quickly determine the answers to those questions.

With Big Pharma's abundant advertising budgets, pharmaceutical reps went even further. They would wine and dine doctors and their teams. In exchange for dispensing more of their drugs, doctors could receive some exciting prizes. Contests were created which included elaborate vacations, cars, cash, etc. Soon, the public started to fall prey to Big Pharma's nefarious agenda. The exact agenda parroted by the medical doctor. Big Pharma masterfully recruited their armies: medical doctors.

Instead of consulting their physiology books, M.D.s began repeating slogans they received from Big Pharma reps to their patients, phrases like: "You are making too much stomach acid. You need this antacid or proton-pump inhibitor." Or, "Your cholesterol is too high at 202. I want to put you on a statin drug because your bad cholesterol is a mess."

Many M.D.s stopped using common sense. They accepted what many of Big Pharma's reps said and instead of checking their medical textbooks or verifying on their own, they acquiesced to writing more scripts. They continued to believe that more drugs were the answer, and as a result, more governing beliefs were formed, such as:

- More vaccines are necessary.
- More flu shots are necessary.
- More antibiotics are necessary.
- Total cholesterol over 180 is dangerous.
- You make too much stomach acid.
- Chiropractors are not real doctors.
- Your diet has nothing to do with Crohn's.
- You need to be on this blood-pressure medication forever.

The broken medical model constantly wielded its power. Their influence began to take root. People began to embrace the "science" being thrown at them. **Collectively, common sense faded away.** Do you think it is a coincidence that coconut oil and a high-fat diet are only now being accepted?

In the early '90s, foods with little or no fat were considered healthy and began flying off the shelves. High-fat snacks such as macadamia nuts were replaced with low-fat snacks such as pretzels.

HEALING VIOLATION #2
The Big Pharma Sales Machine: Profit Before Patients

We have all seen these advertisements, the ones that make you wonder if you have restless leg syndrome or acid reflux or irritable bowel syndrome. These ads encourage the viewer to ask his or her doctor about a specific drug. They suggest that whatever medication is being advertised will quickly take care of your problem. They also indicate that all you have to do to get this medication is ask your doctor — and they are probably right. If you want a quick fix, get the drug.

> **In the United States, prescription drug spending increased 1.3% to $328.6 billion in 2016.** [7]

Many of the advertised medications are for conditions such as hypertension, heartburn, and chronic constipation. These are ailments often remedied when the root cause is addressed. By making appropriate changes in diet, digestion and exercise, positive results occur. Do your M.D.s discuss these options? Of course not.

I'm not saying that *all* drugs are irrelevant. Some drugs actually do help keep people alive. I watched as my own father's health severely declined. He was riddled with multiple cancers and heart disease. Because of the medications and machines, his life was extended for a few short days. When I asked the nurse to turn off all of the IV drips, forced oxygen, etc., I watched my Dad slip away within minutes, literally minutes. Granted, his quality of life while on the medications and machines was non-existent. The point I am making is how the medical model did assist in a process. My family and my Dad's friends had time to gather around him and say goodbye. For that, I will be eternally grateful for medicine. As I have previously stated, in the times of crisis, trauma and emergency care… medicine shines.

The darkness lies elsewhere.

In recent years, the addiction to dangerous pain killers has been in the crosshairs. Many opioid medications like Oxycontin, have come under scrutiny for their careless dispensing and horrific consequences. Who is to blame and at what price?

> **"While lobbying shapes medical policy across the board, it has had a profound impact on the opioid epidemic as deaths quadrupled between 1999 and 2015. The pharmaceutical industry poured resources into attempting to place blame for the crisis on the millions who have became addicted instead of on the mass prescribing of powerful opioids."[8]**

HEALING VIOLATION #3
Fear-Based Doctoring

In my practice, I have seen patient, after patient, after patient taking 10, 12, 18 prescription medications at the same time. When we are talking about Crohn's, colitis, heartburn, there are a lot of meds being prescribed that are harmful and treacherous to the kidneys, liver, gut, etc. This is unacceptable. This is damaging. This is malpractice.

> **"Any doctor will admit that any drug can have side effects, and that writing a prescription involves weighing the potential benefits against the risks."**
> – Mark Udall, former U.S. Senator, Colorado (2009-2015)

A recent study from the Journal of the American Medical Association revealed that nearly 60 percent of Americans today are taking prescription drugs regularly. And 15 percent of Americans are on five or more prescription drugs. This is a greater percentage than any other time in history.

Have these doctors even recommended a nutritional protocol before prescribing drugs aplenty? More startling, perhaps, is just how many patients take whatever their M.D. recommends, to the point of not even knowing what drug they are swallowing.

> **"Researchers found that the prevalence of prescription drug use among people 20 and older had risen to 59 percent in 2012 from 51 percent just a dozen years earlier. During the same period, the percentage of people taking five or more prescription drugs nearly doubled, to 15 percent from 8 percent."[9]**

It is important to understand that the medical curriculum — the whole framework of medical school — is marked with Big Pharma's wily fingerprints. That is a problem. It is a conflict of interest.

The truth is, medical doctors have very little schooling in nutrition. Most of their education is spent on learning the charms of pharmacology.

GUT-Check Goody

"If the U.S. health care system was a country, it would be the 6th largest economy on the entire planet. The losers are the patients; approximately 60 percent of all personal bankruptcies in the United States are related to exorbitant medical bills."[10] - Joseph Mercola, D.O.

Medical students spend ridiculous amounts of time learning about prescription medications. Think about that. In many ways, medical school is an expensive sales training machine for Big Pharma. They are literally learning how to advocate more drugs and help the pig that is Big Pharma to become bigger.

"Besides the many variations on the pill theme, drugstore shelves are packed with an array of breathtaking marvels of pharmaceutical engineering: single-dose, disposable syringes, ointments, eye drops, nasal sprays, medicine-impregnated chewing gum and the ever-more popular transdermal patch."[11] - Jim Hogshire

Further, add the conflict of interest that is the health insurance industry with the above scenario and what you have, my friends, is a license to harm, exclude, damage and kill. This is not what health-care should *ever* be.

Imagine if this much time and effort were actually spent on what truly works and on what heals: food! Food is the real medicine and you will never hear that from the husky trio of terror: Big Pharma, the insurance companies, and the medical doctors. However, fear still seems to prevail because fear is a very powerful emotion. Even with the best of intentions, I have seen many patients thrown off course with these terrible tactics. They are berated with authoritative comments such as, "You have no choice but to take this drug" or "If you do not take this antibiotic you will die," and similar rhetoric.

I want to share something that happened recently in my office. One of my patients complained of his stomach hurting every time he ate. Two or three bites into a meal, he would feel his stomach contracting to the point he could no longer eat anymore. He routinely lost his appetite. He felt nauseous and his mouth would fill with saliva. He would also experience nervousness and anxiety.

When he came to my office, I asked him a few questions. He seemed like a pretty easy case. Based on his symptoms and what he told me about his diet, I gave him two products: a digestive enzyme and a calcium supplement. I sent him home with these 2 simple products (a.k.a. foods).

When he returned two weeks later, he mentioned how fantastic he felt. He could not believe it. His wife could not believe it. He no longer had any of the stomach tension that he experienced before, and now he could happily eat an entire meal. So what did I say? "That's great! This is what I expect. Just let me know if you need me again."

The patient set up a follow-up appointment for two months later. Interestingly, on the day of the appointment, he called to cancel.

Here is why. He went to see his medical doctor and was advised to stop taking the enzyme and calcium supplement. His doctor wanted to put him on medication instead. Even though he was doing well without the medication, and had complete reversal of his symptoms by using food, (the digestive enzyme and the calcium supplement), he was told to stop taking them by his M.D.

Here is the thing, even though the medical approach was ineffective and had previously done nothing for him, he chose to go back to it. Most likely, he started taking an antacid medication, such as a proton-pump inhibitor like Nexium, Prilosec, Protonix, omeprazole, etc. This will prevent his body from digesting protein and absorbing minerals. Because calcium is a mineral, this may adversely affect his bone health, his heart, his muscles, etc. Taking an antacid may also affect his bile, because you need salt for bile, and you need bile to move the bowels. Taking an antacid may also affect his zinc, let's be frank…it may affect everything!

> **"The greatest part of all chronic disease is created by the suppression of acute disease by drug poisoning." – Henry Lindlahr, M.D.**

Did you know these antacids increase stroke risk as well? That is right. Scary stuff. Of course, I can't know for sure what this patient was thinking, but I have to wonder why he would put his faith in something that had not worked in the past, and give up on something that actually was working. Sadly, this case is common. It happens all the time. It has a lot to do with fear. We have been conditioned to have blind faith in the medical model, and to be afraid of any other approach.

Too many people think the medical doctors are indeed more intelligent than any health practitioner on the planet. *(Note: If you feel this way, then you may just want to stop reading now and toss this useless book into the nearest recycling bin.)*

"Drugs never cure disease. They merely hush the voice of nature's protest, and pull down the danger signals she erects along the pathway of transgression." – Daniel H. Kress, M.D.

In order to further this conversation, it is paramount to discuss fear. I can say with certainty that the medical profession has masterfully created a disruption to healing. This is what I like to call "fear-based medicine," the kind of medicine that exposes patients to finger pointing and ridicule if you should dare sport an opinion of your own. If there were one key concept I want you to take away from this book, it is to fully understand that you are the boss of you. You are in control of your body.

I strongly encourage you to ask your doctor better questions. Ask your doctor what *causes* heartburn, what *causes* Crohn's. Ask if there are nutritional solutions to the problem that may be addressed first. I can assure you, heartburn is not a result of a Prilosec shortage in your blood. Crohn's is not a result of a Remicade shortage in your diet. Demand better answers to what nutritional deficiencies exist in your case, or what digestive weaknesses are present. Most illnesses originate in your gut. Do not let fear get the best of you. It is your body. For the most part, you know when something is working and when something is not. Trust yourself. Research more. Listen to your gut. (Of course I mean that literally and figuratively.)

Healing Violation #4
Treating Everyone the Same

Clearly, the medical model is effective when we are referring to situational applications. If you have a broken leg, for example, you need a proper diagnosis and a very clear process of medical treatment. You may need medication to deal with the pain while the bone is reset. There isn't a lot of gray area here. From one patient to another, the issue of a broken leg does not have much variation. For the most part, a broken leg is a similar injury and is going to require comparable treatment.

However, when we are talking about chronic health issues, such as diarrhea, Crohn's, ulcerative colitis, severe heartburn, lupus or other autoimmune illnesses, there is a much greater spectrum for individual treatment that is required. This is especially true if the source of illness is something even more vague or undiagnosed. Chronic digestive issues, general lack of energy, exhaustion, difficulty losing or gaining weight, even feelings of anxiety and depression—these are all stresses that have an origin within the individual. The source varies from person to person; therefore, the treatment should vary from person to person. One thing is for certain, these symptoms and illnesses are clear signs of digestive weakness and energy deficiencies. More on this in later chapters.

This is where the traditional medical model is flawed in gargantuan proportion. Prescription medications do not normalize function. It is impossible for them to do so because they are not foods. In the immortal words of Hippocrates, "Let food be thy medicine and medicine be thy food." Ah, if only the medical profession had maintained this principle at its core over the centuries!

Medications cannot heal the body. The only reason any medication helps with pain is because it effectively blocks enzyme processes in the body. In certain situations, this is necessary and desirable; if there is a major injury, or you are undergoing surgery, for example, this makes sense. Blocking enzyme processes is not something you want to do on a regular basis. Taking drugs will affect *all* the systems in the body. That is why taking one medication often leads to taking *more* medications to deal with the side-effects the original medication created.

You see, only food can heal the body. Foods are fats, carbohydrates, proteins, vitamins, minerals and enzymes. I have worked with so many patients who have found their way back to health using a food-based approach, when they had all but given up on getting any answers or healing from their medical doctors. We need to see people for the unique cases for which they present.

> **"A new scientific truth does not triumph by convincing its opponents and making them see the light, but rather because its opponents eventually die, and a new generation grows up that is familiar with the ideas from the beginning." – Max Planck**

Now, a final note on ego. Why am I able to help people when other doctors are not? To be blunt, it is not because I am special. I would like to think this sometimes, but the honest reason why I get results is quite simple. Aside from the fact that I avoid the aforementioned healing violations, the reason is because I avidly listen and observe my patients. This means really listening and paying attention to each person as an individual. One of the main concerns I have with gastroenterologists is that they treat everyone the same. All patients seem to be a glob of averages.

Everyone has different issues. Even if two people are presenting with the same symptoms, there is no reason to assume that the source of the symptoms is the same in both cases. One person may have an elevated blood pressure because they are severely dehydrated. Another person may experience high blood pressure because they have a fat deficiency. Testing should be customized and very specific to the individual. Physiologically, no two people are exactly the same. If you had a twin, they would most likely test very differently than you would. Each individual is unique in terms of what is causing their particular stress.

Once I shifted my approach in practice, I started seeing instant results. With my G.U.T. Check Protocol, I was effectively helping people by treating them as individuals, which unraveled their particular health mystery.

Even if it repeatedly fails, too often, the broken medical model employs a blanket approach for everyone. Their model operates out of ego, profit, fear and sameness. The good news is, there is a better way.

CHAPTER 3: A Societal Problem

"Your body is a wonderland."
— *John Mayer*

Your body is not only a wonderland but it is also a freaking genius. Seriously! Thank goodness we don't have to think about our heart beating or our lungs filling with air. You don't have to think about your liver making bile or your skin renewing itself over and over again.

As far as I'm concerned, the body's amazing ability to replenish, repair and renew is the most beautiful thing in the universe. We have this innate intelligence, this instinctive natural healing ability. We need to respect and embrace this so much more, like the ancient cultures did.

In the previous chapter, we reviewed four healing violations and the basis of the broken medical model. The goal is to function on such a supreme level that medical intervention is seldom needed. Therefore, let's spend some time reviewing why we get sick in the first place.

As far as I see it, the #1 health-related problem with our society is we judge our health by our symptoms. We think that if we have a sniffle, we're sick. We think if we vomit, we're sick. We think that if we feel great, we're healthy. We think that if we feel well, then we are well. All of these examples are misleading and often untrue.

Now, don't get me wrong, I am all for feeling fantastic. More importantly, I want you to understand the one vital component to true health, and that is health is based on function and not feeling. If you had to choose, it is more important that you function well versus feel well. You cannot judge your health by how you feel. You have to judge your health by how well you function. These are vastly different and extremely important distinctions.

> **"Your body has a miraculous ability to heal itself. In fact, your body is the only healing system that can bring you back into balance when illness strikes."[1] – Hiromi Shinya, M.D.**

Do you want to know something crazy? Sometimes feeling lousy is actually an expression of health.

Let's look closer and discuss how this applies to a fever. When you have a fever, elevated temperatures are necessary to assist in killing excessive foreign invaders. These "bad guys" cannot survive in extreme heat. The body's accurate sensors can indicate when more support is needed. Although a fever may *feel* terrible, the truth is, it is an elegant healing mechanism.

Think of a fever as the body 'sending in the troops.' This healing army refers to your body's immune system, which is rich with specialized white blood cells. Their sole purpose is to search for and destroy any unwanted bacteria or viruses. You want them on that wall. (Yes, I am saying that like Jack Nicholson's role in 'A Few Good Men.')

Pretend you meet up with a bunch of friends and decide on sushi. This place has the tastiest California rolls and their seaweed salads are delicious, too. Two of your buddies order the exact same thing. We will call these two friends Jon and Debra. For the sake of my example, let's just assume the food Jon and Debra ate was equally contaminated with too much e.coli bacteria.

Within an hour of consuming the tainted teriyaki roll, Jon and Debra become violently ill. Thankfully, they live in different houses because both of their toilets are occupied for the next several hours. Both Jon and Debra experienced symptoms of intense vomiting and explosive diarrhea. Now, some of you may think they are sick. But if you consider what is happening here, perhaps you will see that their bodies are actually expressing true health. They feel lousy but their bodies are rigorously removing toxic invaders, and are functioning as they were intended to function — a good thing indeed.

Think of it, would you rather have excessive amounts of e.coli slowly lurking around, wreaking havoc in your body? Or would flushing out the potentially harmful bacteria as soon as possible seem more beneficial? Hopefully, you can see that, although not pretty, it is a much healthier response to rapidly rid the body of toxicity.

Now, I want to give you the other side of the "stress" coin. Let's say you feel fantastic. Does this absolutely indicate pristine health? Does "feeling fantastic" mean you are functioning well? Of course it doesn't. Let me take you through what I mean in this instance. If someone feels fantastic but has clogged coronary arteries, are they truly healthy? Is it possible for the heart to achieve optimal function when arteries are stuffed full of debris?

What if someone feels fantastic but has severe calcium deficiency? Are they healthy? With a deficiency in this vital mineral, is it possible to function properly?

What if someone has a golf ball-sized tumor growing inside of their uterus? Does this exhibit true health? Is it possible for this organ to demonstrate supreme function if it is impaired with such a large mass? Also, would you feel a tumor growing inside the uterus? Of course not.

In each of the above examples, I presented you with the dilemma with which I opened this chapter. That is, you cannot judge your health by how well you feel. You might feel lousy but be expressing optimal health. You may feel fantastic but really be sick. Stop gauging your health *only* by symptoms. Instead, consider paying more attention to how well your body is functioning. Recall two of the Timeless Healing Principles from Chapter 1. One, your body knows how to heal itself. Two: Your body is constantly trying to stay in homeostasis.

Our bodies are always trying to stay alive. Our bodies want to flourish. They are tirelessly working to get to a healthy nirvana. All systems check and recheck. Foreign invaders are effortlessly eradicated. Blood cells recycle themselves for the greater good. Consider this balanced state in all of its grandeur, this desired utopia to be known as **homeostasis**.

GUT-Check Goody

A Disturbing Force

The term, "homeostasis" was first coined in the 1920s by Harvard Physiologist Walter Cannon. "In 1935, Cannon was the first to use the term stress in a non-engineering context. He described stress as "a disturbing force which upsets the person's usual balance."[2]

"Homeostasis refers to a naturally occurring rhythm of the body and its regulatory mechanisms which constantly make dynamic equilibrium adjustments between physiological processes in order to allow us to function consistently in a stable manner. It is a process of ensuring that the internal environment of the body remains within defined normal ranges, and is the set point toward which any change tends to return."[3]

Since we are having an in-depth conversation about stress, we need to acknowledge the work of Austrian Endocrinologist, Hans Selye.

Selye was internationally regarded as one of the world's leading authorities on endocrinology, steroid chemistry, experimental surgery and pathology.

> **"Selye's findings demonstrate that since the human body has its own specific ways of maintaining normal function, and therefore health, any healing attempts should be directed at relieving the stress and providing nutrients for the body to use in it own defense - and its own healing process."**[4] – Howard Loomis Jr., D.C.

Notice the key words "providing nutrients" in Loomis' description. Ask yourself, is the medical model deploying this essential and healing strategy? Are the medications they prescribe nourishing you? Selye later discovered and described the General Adaptation Syndrome. This is a complex explanation of stress. To summarize, when we encounter different stresses, our bodies react in a particular way. The main point to consider is that when under stress, our energy is affected. This then will cause a cascade of negative events to occur. Particularly if the stress is left unchecked.

All the systems of the body are in direct communication with one another. Symptoms, no matter how unpleasant they may be, are signs of stress. Symptoms are signs your body is using to communicate something to you. Are you paying attention? Are you naturally supporting your body's request? Or are you attempting to suppress the symptom with a prescription medication? We'll discuss this more, later.

> **"Almost every health condition, from the common cold to cancer, is directly or indirectly related to stress."**[5] – Donald Yance

It's important to distinguish that there are three main categories of stress. They are:

1. Emotional/Mental Stress
2. Physical/Structural Stress
3. Chemical/Nutritional/Environmental Stress

Examples of **emotional stresses** would include troubles with finances, relationships, divorces, break-ups, anger, anxiety, loneliness, etc.

> **"Digestion, of all the bodily functions, is the one which exercises the greatest influence on the mental state of the individual."** — Jean-Anthelme Brillat-Savarin

Examples of **physical stresses** would include car accidents, sports injuries, slips and falls, carrying a heavy purse on the same shoulder, men sitting on their wallets, the birthing process, etc.

Examples of **chemical/nutritional/environmental stresses** include consuming too much sugar, eating foods that have been sprayed with harmful pesticides and herbicides, excessive alcohol use, food colorings, genetically-modified organisms (GMOs) etc.

According to a nonprofit organization dedicated to protecting human health and the environment, Environmental Working Group (EWG), a study found blood samples from newborns contained an average of 287 toxins, including mercury, fire retardants, pesticides, and chemicals from non-stick products. Of the 287 chemicals, EWG detected in umbilical cord blood, 180 are known to cause cancer in humans or animals; 217 are toxic to your brain and nervous system;

and 208 cause birth defects or abnormal development in animal tests. Clearly, when babies are born loaded with toxic chemicals, it's a sign that toxic exposure is too high.[6]

Each of these stresses or a combination of them is what creates sickness. It is because of these stresses that we lose energy. Stress causes energy deficiencies. Think of it, when your body encounters a stress, it has to account for this deficit. The body will then go about doing all it can to bring you back to balance. When it does this, as you can imagine, additional energy is required. Plus, when stresses accumulate for too long and are not properly addressed, illness and even disease may result.

GUT-Check Goody

Your 365 Hero

"Homeostasis doesn't just happen; it doesn't come automatically. The body is in a constant, 24/7, 365-day-a-year struggle to do this. It follows that every organ system, every tissue in the body, must have adequate nutrition to perform its role in maintaining homeostasis with the extra-cellular fluids — despite ever-changing challenges."[7] - Howard Loomis Jr., D.C.

It is important to point out that of all three categories of stress, emotional stress is the hidden danger in many people. Most do not consider the impact that a life infused with psychological or emotional setbacks cause. In my view, emotional stress is the most traumatic of all forms of stress. The most disturbing part about this is that your body knows no difference from the impact of a head-on car crash versus a divorce. Stress is stress. Either way, your body struggles to maintain homeostasis.

According to the National Cancer Institute, "Psychological stress describes what people feel when they are under mental, physical, or emotional pressure. Although it is normal to experience some psychological stress from time to time, people who experience high levels of psychological stress or who experience it repeatedly over a long period of time may develop health problems (mental and/or physical).

The body responds to physical, mental, or emotional pressure by releasing stress hormones (such as epinephrine and norepinephrine) that increase blood pressure, speed heart rate, and raise blood-sugar levels. These changes help a person act with greater strength and speed to escape a perceived threat.

Research has shown that people who experience intense and long-term (i.e., chronic) stress can have digestive problems, fertility problems, urinary problems, and a weakened immune system. People who experience chronic stress are also more prone to viral infections such as the flu or common cold and to have headaches, sleep trouble, depression, and anxiety."[8]

In my experience working with patients, a lot of their unresolved health challenges stem from emotional abuse from their childhood. It's heartbreaking that so many people have been dealing with this kind of trauma for decades.

> **"Since emotions run every system in the body, don't underestimate their power to treat and heal."** – Candace Pert

Emotions, Pert explains, are not simply chemicals in the brain. They are electrochemical signals that affect the chemistry and electricity of every cell in the body. The body's electrical state is modulated by emotions, changing the world within the body.[9]

> **"Stress causes energy to be deployed for the "stress response," draining the internal life-force energy. Also, when a person is stressed, energy is often diverted away from "protection," which eventually has an impact upon the reproductive hormones, leading to potential problems in reproduction.[10]** – Donald Yance

The complexities of emotional, physical and nutritional stress and their impact on human health is astounding. Thankfully, the Timeless Healing Principles exist. We all have one gland in particular for which to express gratitude: the hypothalamus. Inside your brain, the hypothalamus, measures the different criteria essential to health. Every single second of every day, the hypothalamus is evaluating if you are in a state of stress or a state of health. It is measuring the temperature of your body. It is measuring your blood pressure. It is measuring the concentration of fluids in your body. Your hypothalamus is measuring everything to keep you in a healthy state. This special gland is also communicating to your gut. In turn, the gut is talking back to your brain. There is something dramatically elegant to this healing process. When you see your body as a self-healing organism with all of its brilliance, when you understand the best doctor of all is the one who resides within, you boldly embrace the best secret of all.

"Selye had it right. It all comes down to energy, and nutrition is the key. A stress situation, he observed, will continue without issue as long as the flow of nutrition is maintained and the waste products produced by the affected organs/tissues are transported away and not allowed to accumulate."[11] – Howard Loomis Jr., D.C.

CHAPTER 4: Health Care vs. Sick Care

"Character is a quality that embodies many important traits, such as integrity, courage, perseverance, confidence and wisdom. Unlike your fingerprints that you are born with and can't change, character is something that you create within yourself and must take responsibility for changing." — Jim Rohn

The body is a genuine marvel. Let's discuss how food plays a role. Earlier, I mentioned how symptoms are one of the biggest problems in our society. So too is the prevailing definition of "sick care" versus "health care."

Health care, as we hear it in most media forms, is typically that of sick care, when in fact true health care should be that of prevention and proactive measures.

My homework assignment for you, should you be willing to accept it, is to begin paying attention to the use of this faulty lexicon. When you hear "health care" ask yourself if the term is properly placed. I would bet that more often than not, it is another cloaked misrepresentation of sick care.

Benjamin Franklin is famous for his quote, "An ounce of prevention is worth a pound of cure." How true this resonates today, as it did hundreds of years ago. To take an even closer look, I devised a metaphor that sums up the health care versus sick care philosophy.

Whether it is via my teaching, affectionately known as my "white board action" or when consulting new patients, I deliver the following analogy. I refer to it as the "garbage dump full of rats" visual. I know, it sounds dramatic. Bear with me. This is one of the most effective ways I've found to explain the distinct and polarizing difference between medicine's traditional approach, the sick care model, versus the preventive or functional-based approach to health, the wellness model.

The scenario: Imagine the biggest, nastiest, stinkiest and most polluted garbage dump in all the land. Now, make this example even more ghastly by envisioning gigantic rats dwelling in the infested dump. It is in this "smelly" picture that you will see a clear difference between the medical/sick-care model and the functional medicine/health-care model.

The typical medical doctor's perspective: Most medical doctors will tend to look at a garbage dump full of rats and see the rats as the problem. They will effectively begin the process of destroying, killing and annihilating the rats. To mainstream medicine, the problem here is very much the hairy rodents. Unfortunately, in this example, killing the rats is an after-effect of the initial problem.

Now, on to the typical, functional, wellness-based perspective: The common viewpoint from a functional medicine doctor would be to see the garbage dump full of rats and identify that if it weren't for the gruesome collection of garbage, the rats would not be attracted there in the first place. From a wellness perspective, the problem is very much the garbage. Focusing on the root cause of the problem is essential. In this case, the garbage is the main problem, not the rats. Consider, no more garbage equals no more rats.

In the first example, if one only deals with the rats, without addressing the garbage, eventually more rats will show up. The problem is never fully solved. Sure, rats may disappear for a short time, but until the real problem is taken care of (the garbage) rats will continue to find their way to the garbage dump. Even continuously killing rats does nothing to rectify the situation if the garbage is never removed. Cleaning up and removing the garbage is the solution to make the rats go away.

In my metaphor, the rats are symptoms and the garbage is the authentic root cause or problem.

Rats = symptoms. Garbage dump = the real problem.

Traditional medicine treats symptoms of the original problem whereby functional medicine addresses the root cause. Can you see how chasing after symptoms does nothing to achieve a solution?

If results are important to you, take a step back and evaluate cause and effect. You must identify the source of the stress and focus on removing it. There is no other real solution. If there were only one nugget to take away from my book, let it be this; **ignoring the root cause and chasing after symptoms by throwing dangerous medications at your heartburn, diarrhea, constipation, etc., is futile and potentially dangerous to your health.**

Generally speaking, medical doctors don't take the cause-oriented approach, which is another reason why the medical model is broken. They tend to address symptoms, rather than sources of stress.

Throughout this book, I will be coming from the functional medicine or wellness perspective.

What do you say we move this pertinent metaphor into the realm of human physiology?

I'm here to tell you that cases of inflammation, fatigue, gastrointestinal pain, heartburn, acid reflux, chronic constipation, diabetes, hypertension, etc., are reversible. This is not a broad stroke across the board, but the facts are the facts. The body knows how to heal itself and when you identify the source of stress, which creates the symptoms and sickness in the body, healing happens.

The wellness model is based on the factual understanding that our bodies have incredible healing powers of their own. The very best doctor is the one that resides within you and it is this inner doctor that wants to heal itself. Symptoms are warning lights. Big, flashing, red lights, in fact.

Symptoms themselves are not the problem, just as the rats are not really the problem in our revolting garbage dump analogy. Symptoms are clues. With the right amount of curiosity and commitment, we can follow clues to their root origin or source. Effective treatment as well as lasting results must begin at the source.

The contradiction and the concern is that most Americans are eager to extinguish these guiding clues from our body. Instead of heeding their call, symptoms are seen as insignificant and inconvenient. They are considered bothersome and aggravating. This broad ignorance commences the process of popping the latest pills to cover up the symptoms. Think about it. Imagine if every time you had smoke in your house, you disabled the smoke alarm. Sure, you've gotten rid of the symptom (the annoying alarm) but are you addressing the root cause? Is what you're doing really helping you? Or, imagine that when your oil light goes off in your car, you place a piece of black tape over it and ignore it. Problem solved, right? I can provide multiple, similarly ridiculous examples, but my point is to ask *why are you rejecting your body's exquisite warning system?* A better question would be: **Are you aware of the potential damage you are creating when you cover up cautionary symptoms with harmful prescription medications?**

Because Big Pharma's advertising dollars are so robust, people falsely think the medications are successful and actually healing the body. This couldn't be further from the truth. Too many people blindly take prescription pills without any consideration of their dangers.

Although medications may diminish symptoms for a time, the more significant question is: What effect does this prescription have on the rest of the body? Sure, medicine will cover up symptoms, hence its efficacy. Believe me, I understand when medicine has its place and is necessary. I have often said that when it comes to crisis care, trauma care and emergency care, medications are definitely essential for helping people to stabilize, etc.

But, understand that medications have to be metabolized. They are processed just like everything else you put into your body, from food to water to caffeine to alcohol: through the gut, the liver, the kidneys, the entire digestive system. What effect does dumping medications into the body have? It causes additional strain on your body's systems.

<u>There isn't a medication in the universe that is going to heal and nourish the body.</u>

Therein lies the gigantic problem that faces us. Only nutrition can normalize function.

Taking prescription drugs is not fixing the problem. In fact, what they are doing is dampening or turning off essential body processes while disturbing the body's balance or homeostasis. Taking medications to treat symptoms creates *more* tension and stress on the liver, kidneys, and gut. Medicine isn't going to nourish and heal you. Only food can do that. However, what we have today is a widespread epidemic of over-prescribing medication in cases where the most effective path to healing is going to be a change in diet. This may involve getting the right enzyme therapy, eliminating certain foods from your diet and introducing others. Ultimately, it involves taking responsibility for your overall health.

A Closer Look At Health Care v. Sick Care

<u>Example 1: Fever</u>

If you have a fever, is that a good thing? Is that a sign of health or sickness?

Scenerio: you wake up tired exhausted and with a temperature of 103°.

Typical medical doctor response: "Fever is a sign of sickness." Medical doctors want to suppress the temperature, making you think that you're going to die if you have a fever! (That's the fear mentality that comes from the medical paradigm.)

Typical wellness doctor response: "That's amazing! That's beautiful and brilliant. A fever is a magnificent process that your body has set in place to raise your internal temperature to kill-off the bad stuff. Magical."

Most always, a fever is a beautiful thing.

Example 2: Vomiting

Scenario: Let's say I'm on vacation in a seaside town, and I stop at an oyster bar. I eat six or seven oysters, and they're terrific! Then, I gobble down one more. I realize at the last second that it doesn't taste quite right, but I've already swallowed it. Shortly thereafter, I vomit.

Typical medical doctor response: "You vomited. You will need 2 medications to suppress vomiting and omeprazole. I love dispensing omeprazole. omeprazole is my spirit animal."

Typical wellness doctor response: "You vomited. Awesome, you've removed something that was toxic to your body. Fabulous how the body works, isn't it?"

Example 3: Diarrhea

Scenario: A patient complains of frequent diarrhea.

Typical medical doctor response: "Based on your symptoms and without running any definitive tests, you probably have colitis. I want you on Remicade and antibiotics at once. Here are the prescriptions. Please go fill them now and disregard all of the scary warning signs like blood cancers. Your body is ignorant and needs these medicines. Plus, your condition will never improve. It is something you have to live with. Also, this diarrhea has absolutely nothing to do with your diet. Continue eating whatever you want."

Typical wellness doctor response: "Let's have an appropriate conversation about what has been going on in your life that is contributing to this problem. What have you been eating? What stresses (physical, emotional, nutritional/chemical) have you been under? Your intestines are inflamed. Your liver is under stress and is making thin bile, which is a contributing factor to the extreme urgency you are experiencing."

As you can see, I can be a little playful here, but it truly is no laughing matter. There are two ways to think about health: There is either a wellness model or a medical model.

Keep in mind that when I say medical model, I am excluding crisis care and emergency care. When I say medical model, I am referring to mainstream medicine. I am referring to people going to their medical doctor for some form of symptom or illness like a cold, flu, sinus infection, diarrhea, etc.

The "take-a-pill" method is part of a quick-fix mentality. Today's doctors give pills in too many situations where personal account-ability would be the real answer. If you want a pill for "restless leg syndrome," shouldn't we first address diet? Are you drinking six cups of coffee every morning and eating sugar-laden foods all day long? Could that create symptoms? Of course it could.

Too often, doctors go straight to a pharmaceutical "solution."This is done because it keeps the money circulating. When people focus on self-care, regular exercise, wellness protocols, diet changes, etc., this does not keep money pumping into the powerful pharmaceutical industry.

My question to you is: Are you medically-minded or wellness-minded?

CHAPTER 5: FOOD IS ENERGY

"If you want to find the secrets of the universe, think in terms of energy, frequency, and vibration." — *Nikola Tesla*

Let's define energy. According to Krause's textbook, *Food, Nutrition, and Diet Therapy*, energy is defined as "the capacity to do work. In the study of nutrition, it refers to the manner in which the body makes use of the energy locked in the chemical bonding within food." Other text states, "Energy is a rather subtle property of physical systems that is defined as "the ability to do work." Physicists say "work" is done when a force is applied through some distance. This means that the energy of a system is a property of the system that is able to "make changes happen" through the application of forces.[1]

Your body needs fuel for energy. Like gasoline to a car, our body needs fuel to complete all of the complex functions required throughout our day. As mentioned in previous chapters, although medicine has its place, medicine doesn't heal. Only food heals. Now is the time to discuss how food *is* the real medicine, not drugs.

First, we must begin with one of the biggest misconceptions out there, the phrase: You are what you eat. To be precise, we should instead be saying: You are what you digest.

The caliber of one's overall well-being has everything to do with digestion. You see, just because you're eating a green, leafy salad doesn't necessarily mean your body is receiving the benefits of that salad. When you put food into your mouth, this doesn't guarantee the food is properly broken down for use inside your body.

> **"Life is nourished by food, and the substances in food on which life depends are the nutrients. These provide the energy and building materials for the countless substances that are essential to the growth and survival of living things."[2]**

Think of it this way, before nutrients are distributed throughout your body and to your cells and tissues, food first goes through a tube. This digestive tube or alimentary canal is nearly 30 feet long. It begins at your mouth and ends at your anus. Food enters the mouth, then the esophagus, then the stomach, then the three parts of the small intestines, then the three parts of your colon, then your rectum, then your anus.

> **"The sickest patients often have the best diet."[3] – Howard Loomis Jr., D.C.**

Digestion is so much more than what you eat. "Functions of the alimentary system include receipt, maceration, and transport of ingested substances; secretion of digestive enzymes, acid, mucus, bile, and other materials; digestion of ingested foodstuffs; absorption and transport of products of digestion; and transport, storage, and excretion of waste products."[4]

In order for our bodies to function optimally, we must get most of the food *out of* the tube/alimentary canal and *into* the body. We must digest the food we eat in such a way, that the nutrients reach the cells and provide them with energy. When food is *effectively* digested, our bodies receive energy.

Food is comprised of carbohydrates, proteins, fats, vitamins, minerals and enzymes.

> **"We are made from the chemicals of the earth, which flow through us as we live. We take in food and oxygen, and we give out "wastes" (end products of metabolism) as solids, liquids, and gases. Everything within us and everything we do is sustained by this continual flow of chemicals through our bodies. Apart from oxygen, which we breathe in from the air, all of the chemicals we need are taken in through our mouths as food."[5]**

We need food for three main reasons:

1. It acts as a source of energy, which our bodies require to power all activities, just as cars need the energy released from gasoline to make them run.

2. Our food provides the chemical raw materials that promote the growth and repair of bodily tissues.

3. Some of the chemicals in food serve to regulate vital processes within the body.[6]

Perhaps surprisingly, vitamins and minerals do not supply energy, only macronutrients deliver energy to the body. Let's get a closer look at the role macronutrients (carbohydrates, proteins and fats) play in our body's function, balance and energy. Energy, whether from carbohydrates, proteins or fats, is dispensed to the body's trillions of cells in the form of nutrition.

GUT-Check Goody

Do Vitamins and Minerals Supply Energy?

"When it comes to meeting the body's energy needs, however, vitamins and minerals, while essential, cannot be converted directly into energy. They are building blocks, pure and simple."[7] – Howard Loomis Jr., D.C.

Carbohydrates
First up is carbohydrates. The main role of carbohydrates is to supply energy.

"Most of the energy needed to move, perform work, and live is consumed in the form of carbohydrates."[8]

When it comes to the body's internal energy sequence, it begins with carbohydrates. Always. The body prefers carbohydrates as its primary energy source because carbohydrates easily convert into cellular energy.

If the body experiences low carbohydrate levels for fuel (think of a low gas tank), it must tap into the body's protein reserves for an energy supply. This is accomplished by converting amino acids into glucose. Basically, think glucose = energy.

> "Energy is key. If a person is not able to create an adequate supply of glucose from carbohydrates, the body must get its energy from someplace else. Such patients begin to become protein deficient. This is why patients under chronic stress - be it structural, visceral or emotional - are all protein deficient."[9] – Howard Loomis Jr., D.C.

Please understand, this is not what the body would prefer. The body wants to use carbohydrates as a *regular* energy supply. It is only when this fuel source is depleted that the body will now instruct proteins (amino acids) to deconstruct themselves into useable energy sources (glucose). Think about it, if the body is exhausted of its steady supply of carbohydrate energy drips, and must now convert proteins into energy, can you understand how this will eventually lead to protein deficiency? The body would rather continue using the proteins for their endless tasks such as repairing cells, tissues, organs; creating neurotransmitters such as serotonin and dopamine; building essential compounds such as insulin, thyroxine, and hemoglobin. However, if called upon, proteins must stop what they are doing, so to speak, and energize the body.

Lastly, when this energy depleting cascade continues— in other words, when the body is tanked on carbohydrate *and* protein energy reserves— now the body must tap into fat stores as an energy source. What do you suppose will happen when your body faces deficiencies in utilizing carbohydrates, proteins, and fats as energy supplies? Stress. Symptoms. Sickness. And if unchecked/uncorrected long enough, disease is certainly a possibility. Now ask yourself, is prescription medication a food? Of course not. Therefore, do you see how hurling meds at energy deficiencies creates further stress. toxicity and sickness. Prescription medications *can not* nourish you. Again, only food nourishes you. Only nutrition normalizes function.

> **"It is generally assumed that the consumption of essential nutrients ensures good health, which is not the case when the digestive system has been rendered incompetent by an enzyme-deficient diet.**[10] **- Howard Loomis Jr., D.C.**

GUT-Check Goody

Energy: Food and Survival

"Energy is released by the metabolism of food, which must be supplied regularly to meet the energy needs for the body's survival. Although all energy eventually appears in the form of heat, which is dissipated into the atmosphere, the unique processes within the cells first make possible its use for all of the tasks required to maintain life"[11]

Proteins

If you want to know the power player when it comes to macronutrients, it is protein. Protein is king. Proteins are the healing nutrient. They also provide the body with energy. They are instrumental in growth and repair. They are essential for the body's ability to reach homeostasis. They do it all.

When it comes to proteins, they "perform a major structural role not only in all body tissues but also in the formation of enzymes, hormones, and various fluids and body secretions." In fact, "proteins contribute to homeostasis by maintaining normal osmotic relations among body fluids..."[12]

Let's get back to essential compounds and proteins. Did you know proteins make insulin, thyroxine, hemoglobin, adrenaline, serotonin and dopamine? Proteins also create your antibodies, which are your body's crime fighters. Their role, influence and impact on the body is endless.

"Wherever there is life, whether in plants or animals, enzymes always exist. Enzymes take part in all actions necessary to maintain life, such as synthesis, and decomposition, transportation, excretion, detoxification and supply of energy."[13] - Hiromi Shinya, M.D.

After working with thousands of patients, the biggest disruptor to protein digestion is low stomach acid. Unfortunately, the broken medical model often asserts that "you need antacids because you're making too much acid." *Wrong.* Let's examine the stomach acid and protein connection.

When there is inadequate stomach acid, many problems result. In fact, many people are contributing to their own detriment by willingly taking antacids. Antacids and proton-pump inhibitors significantly disrupt and inhibit protein digestion. You *need* acid in the stomach to digest proteins and to assimilate minerals. As their name implies, antacids or anti-acids turn off the "acid switch." These drugs arrest protein digestion and mineral absorption, thereby disturbing overall gut function such as the reparation, recuperation, and rejuvenation of the body's cells, tissues and organs. It gets worse. Tampering with protein digestion with medicines like Prilosec, Protonix, omeprazole, etc. is a potentially fatal mistake. According to the American Heart Association, these medications may also increase the risk of ischemic stroke.

Your hypothalamus is wicked smart. It is constantly checking body functions. One such function is to detect the presence of food in the stomach. After food enters the stomach, the hypothalamus initiates the process of hydrochloric acid production. The stomach needs this acidic fluid in order to set up the pepsinogen/pepsin conversion required for protein digestion.

> **"PPI's have been associated with unhealthy vascular function, including heart attacks, kidney disease and dementia." - Thomas Sehested, M.D.**

According to a Danish study, overall stroke risk increased 21% among patients who were taking PPI. "At the lowest doses, the authors found either no or minimal increased risk of stroke. At the highest doses they found that stroke risk increased 33% for Prilosec and Prevacid patients, 50% for Nexium patients and 79% for Protonix patients."[14]

What is of little surprise is that when Proctor and Gamble was contacted for a follow-up to the Danish Heart Foundation's study, they replied: "Prilosec is an FDA-approved, safe and effective remedy to relieve frequent heartburn symptoms. Prilosec OTC has the longest history of safe and effective consumer use of any [over the counter] PPI."[15]

When AstraZeneca, the creator of Nexium, was asked to comment on the same study, their response was, "Patient safety is an important priority... and we believe all of our PPI medicines are generally safe and effective when used in accordance with the label."[16]

Ask yourself, is it worth the risk?

In addition, a study in the 'Journal of the American Society of Nephrology' found those who consume PPI's face a 96% increased risk of kidney failure.

Again, I ask you... is your health worth this risk?

Is treating the symptoms of heartburn-related conditions with the stroke-causing and kidney-damaging medications listed above ever going to address the reason or cause of one's heartburn? Of course not. Taking PPI's may be "effective" at removing symptoms but it does so by potentially creating damage elsewhere. Ultimately, heartburn-related issues can be traced back to diet and digestion. Is your M.D. ever discussing this with you? Is your M.D. talking to you about the importance of repairing the mucosal lining and tightening the lower esophageal sphincter? I bet not. When the mucus lining is compromised, symptoms of heartburn may result. When the sphincter that separates the stomach and esophagus is unstable, reflux may occur. Therefore, it is in these areas that repair is needed. Popping Prilosec and the like disturbs protein digestion. Not good.

GUT-Check Goody

The Greeks Said...

"Protein was the first substance to be recognized as a vital part of living tissue. The name was derived more than a century ago from a Greek word meaning "of first importance."[17]

Fats

For far too long, Americans were discouraged from eating a fat-based diet in favor of a high-carb and low-fat diet. Only in recent years, has fat made its overdue and righteous comeback. Fats are needed. They are responsible for making important structures such as: myelin sheaths, phospholipids, cholesterol, prostaglandins, cell membranes, and fatty acids.

Myelin sheaths are sleeves of fatty tissue that protect your nerves. Phospholipids are ingredients inside every cell membrane. Every cell membrane has fat. Cholesterol comes from two main sources: the liver and your diet. It is essential for the formation of your sex hormones, bile salts, etc. You need bile salts to further degrade the fat you are eating. Don't get me started on statin drugs. *Perhaps this will be the topic of my next book.* Prostaglandins stimulate the contraction of smooth muscle and blood vessels. They affect your blood pressure, conception, induction of labor, and nerve-transmission regulation. Fatty acids are smaller components of fats. When one has fatty acid deficiencies, this can lead to dry skin, hair loss, tremors, inability to control blood pressure, inability to conceive or carry a fetus to term, and more. Can you see how fat digestion is significantly relevant to overall health here? Is your medical doctor having a conversation with you about any of this?

GUT-Check Goody

Common Symptoms Linked To Improper Fat Digestion

- Loss of appetite, (especially for meat)
- Frequent sour taste in mouth
- Intolerance of fatty foods or spicy foods
- Pain under the right rib cage
- Frequent constipation

Source: Food Enzyme Institute

When fat digestion is impeded, several body functions are affected. Are you connecting the dots? If carbohydrates, proteins and fats are poorly digested, this leads to compromised body function.

It is paramount that we stop ignoring this.

The inability to digest food (carbohydrates, proteins, fats) leads to stress, symptoms and energy deficiencies. The solution? Understanding that it is *food* that heals. Later, I will review some options that are available to you and always have been.

GUT-Check Goody

Charging Our "Batteries"

"Our cells contain a process for turning fatty acids into glucose. They are processed through a series of chemical reactions called the Krebs cycle. The end result is a rechargeable battery called adenosine triphosphate. (ATP) As ATP provides electrons to keep the cell functioning, it becomes a discharged, rechargeable battery called adenosine diphosphate (ADP). When oxygen is available, for every unit of fatty acids run through the Krebs cycle, we create 38 molecules of ATP. However, if oxygen is unavailable, only 2 molecules of ATP are created for every unit of fatty acids. Thus, as voltage drops, and oxygen levels drop, our metabolism goes from "thirty-eight miles per gallon to two miles per gallon." It is very difficult for cells to have enough energy to function with such inefficient metabolism."[18] - Jerry Tennant, M.D.

Let's talk about what I like to call the quarterback of the gut, which is the liver. The liver is the unsung hero. It's the Rodney Dangerfield organ. It gets no respect for the enormity of its daily tasks. In order to digest fats, you have to have high-quality bile to emulsify fat. Fat digestion is significantly taxing on the human digestive system because it first has to be appropriately prepped for use in the body. Think of it as having to be degreased.

Even in a tremendously healthy individual, there's a significant process that ensues in order to digest fats. There is a lot going on. Fats go through two phases, via the liver, to degrease them for use inside the body. In the process of digesting fats, your body is making free radicals such as hydrogen peroxide. This is potentially very damaging if the body doesn't have enough energy to remove the free radicals.

Important: Healthy biliary function is dependent upon proper stomach acid. Deficient stomach acid, which is extremely common, is going to create thick bile. Thick bile is then going to lead to poor fat digestion. Poor fat digestion is going to lead to poor hormone creation, poor cell membrane creation, poor myelin sheath creation and on and on the cascade goes.

Said another way, low stomach acid will *diminish* the flow of bile. When the flow of bile is lessened, it will cause the existing bile to thicken. With thickened bile, it is common for your stools to be lighter in color and harder to pass. A weakened biliary system will hinder the entire process of fat digestion. Can you understand how this may impact the creation of your myelin sheath, cholesterol, cell membranes, prostaglandins? It is all connected, folks. Food is the real medicine and if we are not digesting food well, I hope you can see how this may lead to significant health issues. Sadly, no medicine in the world is going to address nutritional deficiencies.

Gary L. Wenk, Ph.D., professor of psychology, neuroscience, molecular virology, immunology and medical genetics at Ohio State University stated that diets high in particular types of fat were found to alter basic brain chemistry in such a way that learning was enhanced, age-related cognitive decline slowed and the risk of getting Alzheimer's disease was reduced.

GUT-Check Goody

The Digestion Doc Approved Fats

<u>Examples of healthy fats include:</u>

Avocados
Coconut oil
Egg yolks (from pastured eggs)
Ghee
Grass-fed butter
Nuts
Olive oil
Salmon
Sardines
Sesame oil

Imagine that you have a cell. Each cell needs and requires nourishment. In order for each cell to exhibit supreme function, they need to receive energy. Energy is supplied to the cells to the degree of proper digestion. When food is appropriately digested, cells receive proper energy. The cell energy equation has two components: nutrition coming in and waste going out. Cellular health is directly proportional to the efficiency of these two processes. You cannot have balance if one of these functions is disturbed.

GUT-Check Goody

Raw Materials Are Necessary

"Without the ability to achieve -50mV and the necessary raw materials to make new cells, you cannot maintain your health, and you suffer aging and chronic disease. Our cells are 70 percent water. Thus, as voltage begins to drop, oxygen leaves the cells. This has serious consequences."[19] - Jerry Tennant, M.D.

Dr. Loomis couldn't word it any better when he wrote:

"Does the body have the energy to meet the challenge? That's the bottom line. It's one thing for the brain to send a signal to an organ, and it's quite another thing for that organ to respond. Because that response requires energy. It's at this point that a person begins to experience symptoms, when there's a lack of energy. The symptom is usually a distress signal — an SOS — sent by an organ unable to respond to the brain's instructions due to an energy shortage. The good news is, if you can find the Source of Stress, and give that organ what it needs, you've got it made. The general symptoms of ongoing energy deficiency include: headache, heartburn, indigestion, gas, bloating, infrequent bowel movements, anxiety, irritability, insomnia, etc."[20]

GUT-Check Goody

Keys to Wellness

"Diseases can manifest cellularly, energetically, physically, emotionally, psychologically and spiritually, and will often involve a combination of these causes. Ultimately, to be well you must give love, receive love, and feel a true sense of belonging."[21] - Donald Yance

If your food isn't properly digested, particles of undigested food land in your tissues and joints. This touches off an inflammatory cascade. In practice, I consult with a lot of people who are in the correct weight range and eating all the right foods, yet they don't feel well. This is in part because you are not what you *eat*, you are what you *digest*. Just because the food goes into your mouth doesn't guarantee it goes into your cells.

Undigested food causes symptoms. Many consider these symptoms as part of daily living. This may be true, but what are you doing about it? Although these symptoms are common, it doesn't mean they are normal. If you regularly experience any of the following symptoms or warning signs, your gut is under stress. Remember, your body is trying to tell you something. If there's a problem with digesting food, your body will often let you know in a variety of ways.

I have briefly described what happens with insufficient macronutrient digestion. I have also touched on energy loss as it relates to carbohydrates, proteins, and fats.

Here are the *most common* indications of stress brought on by the inability to digest carbohydrates, proteins, and fats.

Bloating and Gas: Bloating and gas are among the most common symptoms I see in practice. Many patients report feeling bloated every time they eat. This is not normal, and it indicates that your food isn't being digested properly. Frequent and uncontrollable gas is also not normal. Gas is usually an indication of putrefaction. Think of putrefaction as a cauldron of rotting food and noxious chemicals that are slowly decaying inside of you. When this debris exists within your gut, gas and bloat are sure to follow.

Joint Pain: Joint pain typically indicates inflammation and is often the result of a leaky gut. One of the most common causes of joint pain is undigested food. When food is improperly digested, it lands in your tissues and joints and kicks off a cascade of inflammatory responses.

Skin Issues: Skin issues such as eczema, psoriasis and acne are often linked to signs of liver toxicity. When the liver ineffectively processes fats, or when the liver is incapable of digesting fats well, it will push this toxicity out through the skin.

Nausea: Nausea is often a sign your kidneys are taxed. One of the jobs of the kidneys is to clean the blood. If you're getting nausea on a regular basis, even once a month, this is too much. This may suggest your kidneys are overburdened and unable to effectively clean your blood. One of the common sources of kidney stress is also undigested food. In addition, prescription drugs and their harmful chemicals may lead to blood toxicity. Please understand, I am not telling you to stop taking your meds. I'm not a medical doctor. What I am telling you is that medications pollute your blood. Consider how disruptive prescription drugs are to nourishing the body when they contaminate your blood-cleaning kidneys.

Heartburn: Heartburn indicates a compromised mucosal lining and a malfunctioning lower esophageal sphincter. Many are told they have acid-reflux or heartburn-like symptoms because they make "too much" acid. This is physiologically impossible. Instead, it is often the opposite. Most people are not making enough stomach acid.

> **"The drugs with the greatest effect on nutrient absorption are those that damage the intestinal mucosa. Damage to the structure of the villi and microvilli inhibits the brush border enzymes and intestinal transport systems involved in nutrient absorption. The result is general or specific malabsorption of various degrees."[22]**

Diarrhea or Constipation: Diarrhea and constipation are signs that the liver may be under stress. The liver manufactures bile. Bile is necessary for many body functions and one such function is the formation of the stools. In general, if the bile is too thick, constipation is quite common. If the bile is too watery and urgent, diarrhea is likely.

On a cellular basis, the body needs a steady supply of energy coming into the cell not to mention waste to effectively be removed.

Energy is what we get from the food we digest. You do not get energy from prescription medications, and you never will. You only get energy from food when it is adequately consumed and properly digested.

Common Ways Electrons Are Taken from the Human Body (Electron Stealers)

- Acidic water (tap water, chlorinated water, fluoride, most bottled water)
- Carbonated beverages
- Caffeinated beverages (coffee, tea, pop)
- Alcoholic beverages
- Cooked food
- Processed food
- Healers/doctors (when they touch their patients, they lose electrons to patients)
- Hugs (which transfer electrons from one person to another)
- Parent holding a sick child (child gets well quicker, but parent is left tired)
- Moving air (wind, air conditioning, fans, convertibles, and hair dryers)
- Dental infections including root canal teeth
- Heavy metals like mercury, lead, cadmium
- GMO foods
- Fluoride
- Vaccines
- Radiation including x-rays and MRI's
- Chemotherapy
- Most pharmaceuticals [23]

CHAPTER 6: Enzymes: The Sparks of Life

 "Perhaps it would be easier to write about what enzymes do not do, for they are involved in almost every aspect of life."
— Edward Howell, M.D.

It was the fall of 1984. The Detroit Tigers were making a push for the pennant. Life seemed pretty happy. I was only 14 years old. Celebrating a Detroit sports team was simply unheard of. When I was growing up in the seventies and early eighties, our teams were just awful. As far as professional sports go, none of the Detroit clubs were really worth watching. But, it seemed like maybe it was the old English D's year for a baseball dynasty. With each Tiger victory and advancement into the playoffs came elevated school spirit and increased festivities. We were encouraged to wear the Tiger team colors as much as we wanted. You could feel a palpable sense of hope and excitement in the air.

It was incredible to be a kid during that time. People all over Michigan were euphoric in a way I had never seen. It made junior high school fun— all except the part about homework. I tried not to be too distracted with a potential World Series coming to town. School came first. Do you remember the big black science tables that seated 2-4 people? Well, there I was in 8th grade. It was fourth-hour science period with Dr. Charles. On one particular October afternoon, he said something I have never forgotten. We were in the middle of having a group review for an upcoming exam when Dr. Charles said eight specific words which were permanently inscribed into my noggin. It is uncanny now because of my present career, but as I sat there at my ebony desk, I perfectly recall his direct quote. He imparted a secret tip for us. If we were uncertain of an answer come exam day, he offered, "When in doubt, the answer is always enzymes." Huh? To this day, I have no idea why I remembered his words the way I did. I mean, I remember where I was in the room, how I was looking down at my blue Trapper Keeper, the way my #2 pencil was recording his insider info... I remembered his statement as if it were yesterday.

Enzymes: When in doubt the answer is enzymes.

You can imagine how delightful this story is to me now, even decades later.

What I would like to do is share with you why Dr. Charles said these eight words, but more significantly, I will describe how these mighty sparks of life impact everything inside your body. Quite simply, "living things would not be able to sustain life without enzymes." writes Hiromi Shinya in *The Enzyme Factor*.

> **"My theory of how to live a long and healthy life, based on data I have gathered through my decades of medical practice. The data suggests that the entire body and its myriad functions can be understood using one key. That key, the key to a long and healthy life, can be summed up in one word: Enzymes."[1] Hiromi Shinya, M.D.**

Enzymes Are Not Probiotics

First things first. I have to mention that enzymes are not the same as probiotics. So, let's get that cleared up from the jump. Probiotics are bacteria such as lactobacillus acidophilus. Everyone seems to think that probiotics and enzymes are interchangeable. Perhaps this is due to the hefty advertising spend on probiotics these days. When people see a gut-health promo now, they automatically assume: probiotics! Let's "digest" the differences, shall we? Enzymes are sparks of life. Enzymes are special proteins. They are foods. They are catalysts. They are little dynamos. There is nothing in nature or in the body quite like enzymes.

> **"Every cell in the body makes enzymes. They are made in the nucleus." - Howard Loomis Jr., D.C.**

Enzyme research really began back in the 1930s. Eighty years ago, biochemists throughout the world were busy exploring these elegant complexes. At that time, scientists were able to identify 80 different enzymes. Today, it is estimated that more than 5,000 enzymes have been discovered.

Dr. Edward Howell was the leading pioneer in the field of enzyme nutrition.

"Dr. Edward Howell received his medical degree in 1924. He worked at the Lindlahr Sanitarium where individuals suffering from exhaustion were treated with a regimen of exercise, hydrotherapy, manipulation, outdoor exposure and a raw vegetarian diet. It was during this time that the medical community was beginning to recognize the impact of canning and processing on human health and wellness. The processes significantly reduced the vitamin and mineral content of fruits and vegetables creating a need for supplementation. Dr. Lindlahr created a vitamin supplement that his patients could use when they ate cooked, canned or processed foods. Young Dr. Howell observed that patients who ate the raw foods had greater vitality and wellness than those who consumed cooked foods even with the vitamin supplement. He concluded that something present in the raw food other than vitamins and minerals played a vital role in maintaining human health. His passionate search for this vital force led him to discover the presence of food enzymes and their role in human health and longevity."[2]

Howell "was the first researcher to recognize and to outline the importance of enzymes in food to the nutrition of human beings. He wrote *The Status of Food Enzymes In Digestion and Metabolism* in 1946. It took him more then 20 years to complete *Enzyme Nutrition*, which is a condensed version. The original work has about 700 pages, is approximately 160,000 words long and contains 695 references to the world's scientific literature, as well as 47 tables. It contains the reference and source materials for Dr Howell's enzyme theories, which he called the "Food Enzyme Concept." The book reviews the scientific literature through 1973."[3]

Howell describes enzymes this way:

> **"I define the enzyme complex in biological rather than chemical terms. The enzyme complex harbors a protein carrier inhabited by a vital energy factor ... Thought of for years as catalysts, enzymes are much more than these inert substances. Catalysts work by chemical action only, while enzymes function by both biological and chemical action. Catalysts do not contain the 'life element,' which is measured as a kind of radiation which enzymes emit."[4] -Edward Howell, M.D.**

Despite my devotion to enzyme nutrition, those who came before me say it better than I ever could. As far as I'm concerned, Dr. Howell's and Dr. Loomis' work should be recognized for its outstanding contribution to gut health, digestion, and longevity. I have chosen to deliver the best information in the most concise way by including numerous quotes, bullets, etc. throughout this chapter.

There are three classes of enzymes:

Food Enzymes
Digestive Enzymes
Metabolic Enzymes

Food Enzymes
Enzymes are a natural component of raw foods and play a vital role in digestion. These enzymes have been termed "food enzymes".
• Food enzymes digest foods in the upper stomach prior to inactivation by gastric acid secretion. This is often termed

"pre-digestion,"

- Food enzymes are destroyed by the heat associated with cooking, canning, pasteurization and other food processing techniques.

In the absence of dietary food enzymes, the body is forced to secrete more enzymes, acid and bile to deal with the increased digestive burden. The ability of the body to modulate the secretion of enzymes based upon its digestive needs has been termed "adaptive secretion."

The increased digestive burden robs the body unnecessarily of energy and resources which contributes to degenerative disease. Supplemental enzymes replace the enzymes lost in cooking and processing. Fungal and plant enzymes work in the upper stomach in the process of pre-digestion. Neither enteric coated enzymes nor pancreatic supplements are able to work under those conditions and do not contribute to pre-digestion.

The consumption of food enzymes as well as supplemental enzymes, prevent/reduce the occurrence of Digestive Leukocytosis (inflammation that occurs after the consumption of cooked foods). Food enzymes and supplemental enzymes may be absorbed and may elicit systemic effects.[5]

Digestive Enzymes

The second category is the digestive enzymes, of which there are about 22 in number. Most of these are manufactured by the pancreas. They are secreted by glands in the duodenum (the upper part of the small intestine) and work to break down the bulk of partially digested food leaving the stomach.[6]

Digestive enzymes have three main jobs: the digestion of proteins, carbohydrates, and fats. **Proteases** are the enzymes that digest proteins. **Amylases** are the enzymes that digest carbohydrates. **Lipases** are the enzymes that digest fats. It is important to point out that during the digestive process, a protein enzyme or protease can only digest proteins. A protein enzyme cannot digest a carbohydrate or a fat. A carbohydrate enzyme such as an amylase can only digest a carbohydrate. It cannot digest a protein or a fat, and so on. This is why it is so essential to discover where your area of macronutrient weakness is. If you're interested in my Leaky Gut Test Analysis and Digestive Stress Profile, you can discover more about this unique testing process by visiting www.gutprotocol.com. In the last chapter, I will also review my proprietary GUT-Check Protocol.

When it comes to those powerful warning signs and symptoms, have you considered the damaging role undigested food plays?

GUT-Check Goody

Your Protective Barrier

"Food particles not digested well enough to be absorbed across the gut wall, mostly proteins and sugars, are acted upon by unfriendly bacteria in the last section of the small intestine (the ileum) and in the colon. The result is an overgrowth of unfriendly bacteria and the toxins they release, along with the accumulation of undigested food in the large intestine. The more putrefaction that is taking place, the more constipated a person becomes. Toxic chemicals, including indican, are formed. These chemicals can irritate the mucosal barrier that protects the wall of the gastrointestinal tract. When the mucosal barrier is sufficiently compromised, the result is "leaky gut" syndrome. The integrity of the bowel itself becomes compromised in leaky gut syndrome, allowing partially-digested food particles and bacterial endotoxins to leak through the gut into the lymphatics and the bloodstream. These compounds can cause a number of inflammatory problems before they can be detoxified by the liver and eliminated. They can overwhelm weaker organs, producing pain and an inflammatory immune response. This is why the body's ability to produce and maintain normal, healthy, well-nourished mucosal cells, to protect the walls of the gastrointestinal tract, is imperative."[7]

- Howard Loomis Jr., D.C.

Metabolic Enzymes

Next up are metabolic enzymes. They are the largest of the three enzyme classifications. Metabolic enzymes involve all bodily processes including breathing, talking, moving, thinking, healing, and operating the immune system.

> **"Our bodies — all our organs and tissues— are run by metabolic enzymes. These enzyme workers take proteins, fats and carbohydrates (starches, sugars, etc.) and structure them into healthy bodies, keeping everything working properly."**[8] - Edward Howell, M.D.

Additionally, metabolic enzymes neutralize poisons, carcinogens, pollutants, tobacco smoke, DDT, etc. They then change these toxic chemicals into less corrosive configurations so that the body can efficiently eliminate them.

> **"Hundreds of metabolic enzymes are necessary to carry on the work of the body - to repair damage and decay, and heal diseases."**[9] - Edward Howell, M.D.

The Supremacy of Raw and Fermented Food
If there is one thing you could immediately implement to improve digestion and to prevent degenerative diseases brought on by eating cooked and processed foods, it is to eat more raw and fermented foods. For thousands of years, ancient cultures have incorporated these enzyme-rich foods because of their comprehensive health benefits.

> **"Nature has enclosed all raw foods with the correct and balanced amounts of food enzymes either for human consumption or eventual decomposition outside the human body."**[10] - Edward Howell, M.D.

Almost all traditional societies incorporate raw, enzyme-rich foods into their cuisines—not only vegetable foods but also raw animal proteins and fats in the form of raw dairy foods, raw fish and raw muscle and organ meats.

These diets also traditionally include a certain amount of cultured or fermented foods, which have an enzyme content that is actually enhanced by the fermenting and culturing process. The culturing of dairy products, found almost universally among preindustrialized peoples, enhances the enzyme content of milk, cream, butter and cheese. Ethnic groups that consume large amounts of cooked meat usually include fermented vegetables or condiments, such as sauerkraut and pickled carrots, cucumbers and beets with their meals. Even after being subjected to heat, fermented foods are more easily assimilated because they have been predigested by enzymes. In like manner, cooked meats that have first been well aged or marinated present less of a strain on the digestive mechanism because of this predigestion.[11]

The enzymes found in raw foods help begin the digestive process. This reduces the body's need to produce digestive enzymes. Specifically, food enzymes present in raw foods initiate the process of digestion in the mouth and stomach.

> **"Fermented foods and aged foods are predigested by their own inherent enzymes or by starters such as those often used in production of sourdough bread, yogurt, and some cheeses."[12] - Edward Howell, M.D.**

Dr. Howell found that "a diet composed exclusively of cooked food puts a severe strain on the pancreas, drawing down its reserves, so to speak. If the pancreas is constantly overstimulated to produce enzymes that ought to be in foods, the result over time will be inhibited function. Humans eating an enzyme-poor diet, comprised primarily of cooked food, use up a tremendous amount of their enzyme potential in the outpouring of secretions from the pancreas and other digestive organs. The result, according to the late Dr. Edward Howell, is illness and lowered resistance to stress of all types. He points out that humans and animals on a diet comprised largely of cooked food have enlarged pancreas organs while other glands and organs, notably the brain, actually shrink in size.[13]

> **"Many if not all degenerative diseases that humans suffer and die from are caused by the excessive use of enzyme-deficient cooked and processed foods."[14] - Howard Loomis Jr., D.C.**

If you didn't have an idea of how powerful and essential enzymes are to human digestion, I hope after reading directly from the greats themselves, your perception has shifted toward incorporating enzyme nutrition into your life. Dr. Howell stated, "the length of life is inversely proportional to the rate of exhaustion of the enzyme potential of an organism." Take heed. Now, consider yourself aware of one of the most insider healing practices. Enzymes. These sparks of life have dramatic responsibilities to keeping your health in balance.

Key Takeaways By Edward Howell, M.D.

"Enzymes are substances that make life possible. They are needed for every chemical reaction that takes place in the human body."

"Our enzyme potential has a problem similar to a checking account which could become dangerously deficient if not continually replenished."

"No mineral, vitamin, or hormone can do any work without enzymes."

"Enzymes also aid in converting the prepared food into new muscle, flesh, bone, nerves, and glands."

"They also assist the kidneys, lungs, liver, skin, and colon in their important elimination tasks."

"Every organ and tissue has its own particular metabolic enzymes to do specialized work. One authority made an investigation and found 98 distinct enzymes working in the arteries, each with a particular job to do."

"The length of life is inversely proportional to the rate of exhaustion of the enzyme potential of an organism. The increased use of food enzymes promotes a decreased rate of exhaustion of the enzyme potential."

"The primary appearance of enzymes was inseparably connected with the appearance of life. We cannot repeat the process in the same way as it occurred in nature since it required billions of years to take place."

"...nearly half of our daily production of protein in the body consists of enzymes."

"...each of us, as with all living organisms, could be regarded as an orderly integrated succession of enzyme reactions."

"Nature's plan calls for food enzymes to help with digestion instead of forcing the body's digestive enzymes to carry the whole load."

"Even thinking involves some enzyme activity."

"The most potent digestive enzymes secreted by the human body are amylase and protease. In fact, "the pancreas is the biggest factory devoted to turning out digestive enzymes. The pancreas receives enzyme precursors from the body cells or the bloodstream and supplies the finishing touches."[15] *Enzyme Nutrition*

Bonus GUT-Check Goodies

GUT-Check Goody

Protein Power

"Food enzymes include proteases for digesting protein, lipases for digesting fats and amylases for digesting carbohydrates. Amylases in saliva contribute to the digestion of carbohydrates while they are being chewed, and all enzymes found in food continue this process while it is mixed and churned by contractions in the stomach. The glands in the stomach secrete hydrochloric acid and pepsinogen, which initiate the process of protein digestion, as well as the intrinsic factor needed for vitamin B12 absorption; but the various enzymes needed for complete digestion of our food are not secreted until further down line, in the small intestine. However, while food is held in the stomach, the enzymes present in what we have consumed can do their work before this more or less partially digested mass passes on to the enzyme-rich environment of the small intestine."[16]

GUT-Check Goody

Dead at 118°

"All enzymes are deactivated at a wet-heat temperature of 118 degrees Fahrenheit and a dry-heat temperature of about 150 degrees. It is one of those happy designs of nature that foods and liquids at 117 degrees can be touched without pain, but liquids over 118 degrees will burn. Thus, we have a built-in mechanism for determining whether or not the food we are eating still contains its enzyme content."[17]

GUT-Check Goody

Nutty Inhibitors

"Grains, nuts, legumes and seeds are rich in enzymes, as well as other nutrients, but they also contain enzyme inhibitors. Unless deactivated, these enzyme inhibitors can put an even greater strain on the digestive system than cooked foods. Sprouting, soaking in warm acidic water, sour leavening, culturing and fermenting-all processes used in traditional societies-deactivate enzyme inhibitors, thus making nutrients in grains, nuts and seeds more readily available."[18]

GUT-Check Goody

Exceptional Plant Foods

"Most fruits and vegetables contain few enzymes; exceptional plant foods noted for high enzyme content include extra virgin olive oil and other unrefined oils, raw honey, grapes, figs and many tropical fruits including avocados, dates, bananas, papaya, pineapple, kiwi and mangos."[19]

GUT-Check Goody

Raw Honey and Amylase

"Raw honey is noteworthy for having considerable plant amylase. The amylase does not come from the bee but is a true plant enzyme, concentrated from the pollen of flowers."[20] - Edward Howell, M.D.

CHAPTER 7: GUT-Check Protocol

"Those who do not find time everyday for health must sacrifice a lot of time one day for illness." — *Father Sebastian Kneipp*

He came running up the stairs. He was panicked and out of breath. This wasn't to be expected from a man in his early 50s. What he said next, forever changed me. He cried out that he had just lost control of his bowel movement. There he was, in the driveway of his home, somewhere safe, somewhere close, but it didn't matter. He didn't make it in time.

Many often ask me what made me get into this line of work as The Digestion Doc. What made me choose to help people regain their freedom from the crappiest, yes crappiest, health conditions like Crohn's, ulcerative colitis, etc.? Well, the short answer is to help them restore their freedom. My most sacred value has been and always will be freedom. The more distinctively personal response as to why I do this refers to the above story.

The man whose most-humiliating experience I witnessed second-hand is my uncle. It was 1996, I was visiting my grandmother. My uncle had just left to run an errand. He was out of the house for no more than 15-minutes when his urgent consequence facilitated his return. I will never forget his frantic words, his embarrassment, his dismay... It is one of those things you wish you could undo.

Having said that, I recognize this was a moment that attached purposeful intention within me. I thought, if there is anything I can ever do in my career to help people conquer this horrible and unpredictable digestive problem... if I could provide relief and comfort so people could stop fixating on bathroom locations and packing extra changes of clothes, then I would readily accept this task.

What took me by surprise in practice was just how many people's stories resembled that of my uncle. There are thousands of digestive chronicles I could share. No matter the story, the collective point is to find out why this is happening to the individual, and nourish the body back to health. We need to live our best lives, and if our health is forcing sacrifices and disappointing circumstances on us, we need to pay attention as to why this is.

Now, I want to detail eight specific reasons why one may have digestive complaints. I refer to them as the **Eight Phases of Digestive Stress**. I learned this sequence from my mentor, Dr. Loomis. As our digestion becomes stressed, more areas of the body are affected.

The 8 Phases of Digestive Stress are:

1. Diet
2. Digestion
3. Bowel Movements
4. Inflammation
5. Immune System
6. Autonomic Nervous System
7. Endocrine System
8. Lymphatic System

Regarding our health, diet is the first place in which one's digestion is stressed. Digestive stress may then impact bowel movements, and so on. In this cascade, the easiest to reverse is diet, or phase one. The most difficult to reverse is lymphatic stress, or phase 8. Now, I will supply my take on these 8 phases and dig-in with more detail as to what I see in practice and how it may assist you.

Phase One: Diet

If you are brand new to me, I would like to reveal one of my favorite hashtags, **#PPCSW**. Each letter in this tag represents 5 foods that I highly recommend you avoid and/or eat on rare occasions only. I refer to these five foods as the "**Five Belly Busters.**" I have selected these particular foods because they repeatedly show up as the culprits in many patients' digestive complaints. Whether it is gas, bloating, cramping or diarrhea, you may be experiencing, I am fairly certain you consumed a belly-buster ingredient. The belly busters consist of pork, peanuts, corn, soy and wheat. If you are having any modicum of digestive discomfort and if you are discovering me for the first time, here is some important and simple advice: avoid these foods for a solid two weeks, and watch how much better you feel.

Up first, Pork. The first P in **#PPCSW** is genetically similar to humans. When we utilize their hearts, their heart valves, their hormones, etc., they effectively work inside the human body. When we eat their tissue, you probably can deduce where I am going with that. If you have any measure of a loose stool, whether it's Crohn's, diarrhea, IBS, I would absolutely recommend you *avoid* pork.

When George Orwell wrote in his classic novel *Animal Farm* that man and pig are almost identical, he was closer to the truth than he realized. Scientists have undertaken the largest study of the pig genome and have found that swine are adaptable, easy to seduce with food, and susceptible to domestication — much like humans. The findings, published in the journal, *Nature,* also show that pigs suffer from the same genetic and protein malfunctions that account for many human diseases, including Alzheimer's, Parkinson's and obesity.[1]

Number two on my list of belly busters stands for P or peanuts. Peanuts have a mold that grows on their shell called aflatoxin.

"Aflatoxins are a family of toxins produced by certain fungi that are found on agricultural crops such as maize (corn), peanuts, cotton-seed and tree nuts. The main fungi that produce aflatoxins are Aspergillus flavus and Aspergillus parasiticus, which are abundant in warm and humid regions of the world. Aflatoxin-producing fungi can contaminate crops in the field, at harvest and during storage."[2]

Due to the humid climate of the American southeast, mold grows. As peanut butter is processed, this mold gets scraped off of the shells and into the nut butter. Peanuts grown in New Mexico or dry climates are better options. An example would be valencia peanuts.

Number three on my list of belly busters stands for C or corn. Number four on my list of belly busters stands for S or soy. Both corn and soy are on the list because they are commonly genetically modified.

What is a GMO?
Genetically modified organisms (GMOs) are living organisms whose genetic material has been artificially manipulated in a laboratory through genetic engineering. This creates combinations of plant, animal, bacteria and virus genes that do not occur in nature or through traditional crossbreeding methods.

Most GMOs have been engineered to withstand the direct application of herbicide and/or to produce an insecticide. However, new technologies are now being used to artificially develop other traits in plants, such as a resistance to browning in apples, and to create new organisms using synthetic biology. Despite biotech industry promises, there is no evidence that any of the GMOs currently on the market offer increased yield, drought tolerance, enhanced nutrition, or any other consumer benefit.[3]

As far as corn is concerned, if you can find a non-GMO corn chip, that's a better and far safer option. As for soy, I am not a fan. Soy has been known to mess with endocrine systems of the body and it also robs the body of important minerals such as zinc.

Number five on my list stands for W or Wheat.

For those playing along, wheat products *also* include white flour. White flour is simply refined wheat flour. I appreciate that this is the hardest for most to cut out, but understand the reason I recommend removing it is because the crops have been altered and changed, as well.

Those are the five belly busters. Pork, peanuts, corn, soy, wheat #**PPCSW**. In the near 20 years in practice, these are the foods that regularly cause trouble. They are the common denominators or the repeat offenders.

When it comes to growing healthy foods so that our diets can flourish, we need to be mindful of a few other points. The American government advocates for corporate farming practices and concentrated animal feeding operations (CAFOs). This usually means faster production and less-healthful products. Not good.

Bottom line, big agricultural giants are all about profit. They have an ungodly amount of money, reach and influence. Just as Big Pharma is quite connected in the American congress, you better believe there is a lot of money changing hands with politicians and big agricultural and biotech seeds as well.

"Some anti-GMO activists, including Indian scientist and organic-farming champion Vandana Shiva, have blamed the high suicide rates directly on biotech seeds—specifically, cotton tweaked by Monsanto to contain the Bt pesticide, now used on more than 90 percent of India's cotton acreage. Shiva has gone so far as to declare them "seeds of suicide," because, she claims, "suicides increased after Bt cotton was introduced."[4]

Let me interject a critical point. Since we are talking about digestive stress, I want to talk to you about hydration. Did you know we can go weeks without food? The same is not true when it comes to water. In fact, we cannot last long without water. It's essential that you're getting close to 96 ounces of water per day. Clearly this is a variable for every person. Don't *try* to drink water. *Just do it!* It really is that essential.

The Essential Functions of Water

"Whether to improve the flow of the gastrointestinal system or the flow of blood and lymph fluids, water has very broad functions in the body."

"Water has many function's inside the human body, but the biggest function is to improve blood flow and promote metabolism. It also activates the intestinal bacterial flora and enzymes while excreting waste and toxins."

"It carries out the important functions of purifying, filtering, and transporting excess water, proteins, and waste through the bloodstream."

"Inside the lymph vessels are antibodies called gamma globulins, which have immune functions and enzymes called lysozymes that have antibacterial effects."

"In order for the immune system to function properly, good water is absolutely necessary."

"Water is vital to all parts of the body. A body cannot sustain itself without adequate water. That is the reason why plants do not grow in the desert."

"In a human being, if water is not distributed properly, that person will not only become malnourished, but waste and toxins will also accumulate inside the cells, unable to be excreted. In the worst-case scenario, the accumulated toxins will damage cell genes, causing some cells to become cancerous."

"Providing nourishment to and receiving and disposing of waste from the body's 60 trillion cells are microfunctions of water. These microfunctions, which produce energy and break down free radicals, also involve many enzymes. In other words, if water is not precisely distributed to all 60 trillion cells, enzymes will not be able to sufficiently accomplish those functions."

"In order for enzymes to work properly, not only are various trace nutrients such as vitamins and minerals needed, but they also require the medium in which these things are transported, namely, water."[5] - Hiromi Shinya, M.D.

Phase Two: Digestion

Remember that the phrase, "you are what you eat" is false. Better stated, it should be: **"you are what you digest."**

There is quite a difference between these two statements. Most of the patients I work with are actually consuming a fairly clean and healthy diet, but they feel terrible. Keep in mind the feeling/function discussion from Chapter 3-4. Symptoms are warning signs. Please pay attention to them! Quieting symptoms with prescription medications may offer a temporary patch but it is not the nourishing answer. Also, never forget how well you function is of critical significance for digestive health.

Digestion is really summarized into two big things:

1. How well you convert the food you are eating into proper, usable nutrition.

2. How well you eliminate waste.

Phase Three: Bowel Elimination

Let's move into the third phase of digestive stress which is bowel elimination. I specialize in helping patients with Crohn's, ulcerative colitis, constipation, diarrhea, etc. It is imperative that we discuss what a healthy bowel movement should look like. Here is my best description for you. Let's do it.

The perfect bowel movement should go something like this: You're recently up and about. You get up from your night's sleep and within an hour of rising, you have a bowel movement. Or maybe you're walking around during your day, or you're at work, or you're doing whatever... when all of a sudden your brain gently says, I need to eliminate waste. Notice my use of the word "gently". This is intentional of course because you should have absolutely no urgency to have a bowel movement. You should be able to "hold it" if you needed to.

Anyway, back to the perfect bowel movement. You go into the bathroom and you sit down and you're doing your deal, and within 90 seconds or less comes a stool that is Hershey chocolate brown and the shape of a log or a torpedo. This stellar stool should be well-formed and it should not dirty the toilet water or break apart when you flush. In fact, since I am painting the picture of the perfect poo, there should also be a point at the end of your stool. This is a sign your "cutter" is working correctly. As your stool makes its relieving exit, and when you wipe, there should be little to zero residue on the toilet paper. I refer to this wiping wizardry as the "clean sweep". Now, if you're still reading after such doodie descriptors, well congratulations because that is the perfect bowel movement. You should move your bowels 1-4 times per day, every day. Are you ready for another interesting doo-doo detail?

Your stool should actually have a slightly sweet-smelling odor to it. You'll know what I'm talking about when you have this bowel movement. Sadly, I am willing to bet many of you have never experienced this kind of bowel movement. If you catch a whiff in most public bathrooms, you will know that a lot of peoples' bowel movements are in rough shape. I am shocked at the sensory smack I get when walking into an airport bathroom. These are some very digestively disturbed people. I mean, a lot is going wrong in their gut for their bm's to smell that ghastly.

Let's review. A perfectly formed stool should resemble a log or a torpedo. It does not have to be the shape of an S, like Doctor Oz says, I don't even know where he gets that. Your stool should be dark brown. Think of a Hershey chocolate bar as a good gauge. Your stool should be so well-formed that it does not break apart when flushed.

Quick tip: look at your stool. If you're not, you should be because looking at your bowel movements is a great indicator of how healthy or sick may be. As an example, if your stools are always the shape of pebbles, then you are constipated. If your stools usually float, then you're not properly digesting and/or metabolizing fats. If you would like more information on form, I recommend you review the Bristol Stool Chart.[6]

Even though we are thoroughly examining what constitutes a perfect bowel movement, I have another bonus tip I want to throw in here. I highly advise you to analyze your urine color before flushing. You should remember from a few paragraphs back that digestion is the combination of breaking down food for appropriate use as well as properly eliminating waste. Your urine is also an integral element of elimination. Do not focus *only* on stool, you need to view both your stool and urine on a daily basis.

What you are eliminating really leaves clues. Upon rising, your first urine should be the darkest color. This is because you are expelling waste and acids. Throughout your restful slumber, your body was hard at work removing toxins and debris. Your first urination is going to be a dark yellow-orange color. As you slept for numerous hours, your body metabolized debris, poisons, toxins, etc. In addition, your urine is darker in color because of the acid accumulation. When we sleep, we are not breathing deeply or correctly so there is a build up of carbon dioxide, which is an acid.

It is for these reasons that your urine is that dark yellow, orange color. Amazing, right? As your day ensues and as you hydrate, your urine should lighten in color throughout the day. There should barely be a yellow color to it at all. Your urine should be nearly clear in color. However, if you notice your urine remains dark yellow-orange throughout the day, this is not healthy. You are likely dehydrated. If this is you, please go back and review the section on the Essential Functions of Water.

Also, keep in mind that certain supplements such as B-complexes make the urine a bright yellow color. If you are not taking any supplements but you have the dark yellow-orange urine, begin increasing your water intake. Remember, I suggest you to hit the 64-96 ounce mark each day. As your day progresses, and as you hydrate effectively, you should see a clearer, water-like appearance to your urine's color. If your urine is really foamy, that is often indicative of dehydration, and fat/protein digestive issues.

You need to be your best health advocate. You are the 5-star general of your body. No one else. If you don't pay attention to these simple clues, who will?

Phase Four: Inflammation

The fourth phase of digestive stress is inflammation. Remember, the further into the 8 phases we go, the more stressed you are. As for inflammation, there are three stages involved.

Stage 1: the acute/protection phase. This stage occurs at the very beginning. As an example, when you break your arm. This is the first 72 hours. This period of inflammation involves, swelling, bracing, and protection.

Stage 2: The second stage of inflammation is the repair phase. This period will last from 72 hours to six weeks. This is the collagen rebuilding phase. Special tip for all of the bone broth lovers out there, make sure you're eating enough vitamin C while consuming your broth as vitamin C helps to make collagen. I recommend incorporating more red bell peppers into your diet because they are a spectacular source of vitamin C as are lemons.

Stage 3: The third and final phase of inflammation is the remodeling phase. This stage takes the longest. Expect a healing period of 3 weeks to 2 years. Although this stage takes the longest, remember the body's brilliance. This time is required to help restore balance.

When we discuss inflammation, whether that is in a joint, a muscle group, or the gut, there are five cardinal signs. These signals include redness, pain, heat, swelling, and loss of function.

Typically, people think of inflammation and consider a finger sprain, or a back strain, or something of this nature. Now, I want to challenge you to think about inflammation with respect to your digestion. Imagine what redness, pain, swelling, or loss of function may look like inside your entire gastrointestinal tract?

Do you suppose the cramps, or abdominal discomfort may be rooted in inflammation?

Is it possible your painful and uncontrollable gas and bloating originates from an inflammatory process?

In fact, would you be surprised if I told you the biggest cause of inflammation is **undigested food**. Don't be alarmed if you didn't think this was a possibility, you are definitely not alone there. Most people never recognize the significant damage undigested food can cause.

The simple truth is if you are not properly breaking down the fats, the carbs, the proteins, the vitamins and the minerals from your meals, you likely have inflammation. I want to take you on another visual journey. This time, I want you to imagine big pieces of undigested food that are floating or flocculating throughout your bloodstream. These undigested food particles are too large to get inside the cell. They simply cannot pass because the cell membranes are designed in such a way that only compounds with a special size or chemicals that have a special key can get in. We have all seen dust accumulate in our houses. Now, think of this dust but imagine it is of a food variety. Pretend you have food dust floating around in your body. Where can it possibly go? The answer is in your tissues and joints. This is where the undigested food settles. As for symptoms that result, think stiff, achy joints, headaches, heartburn, diarrhea, constipation, mental anguish, forgetfulness, brain fog, anxiety, candida, bad breath, etc. You can literally name a symptom and the chances are high that it can be linked to undigested food.

Phase Five: Immune System

A quick recap. Diet, digestion, bowel movements, inflammation. We've gone through the first four phases. Now, we're on number five, which is your immune system. What I want to just quickly say here is 80 to 90% of your immune system lives in your gut.

> **"The human body needs food enzymes to predigest foods. When food enzymes are not present, the body must mobilize the immune system to complete the digestive process and clean up the resulting toxic mess." - Howard Loomis Jr., D.C.**

If we're not heavily focusing on digestive health, then we are ignoring what's happening with the immune system.

What stresses the immune system more than anything?

Answer: *Undigested food.*

Once homeostasis is compromised, you will see symptoms.

Pick a symptom:

Fever, Redness, Swelling, Pain, Headaches, Heartburn, Nausea, Bloating, Gas, Constipation, Diarrhea, Abnormal Motion, Depression, Panic Disorder, Fatigue, Sore Joints, and so on.

Not only are these signs of compromised immune function, but they are also cardinal signs of inflammation and enzyme deficiency. Our immune system is essential for our survival. Without an immune system, our bodies would be open to attack from bacteria, viruses, parasites, and more. It is our immune system that keeps us healthy as we drift through a sea of pathogens.

This vast network of cells and tissues is constantly on the lookout for invaders, and once an enemy is spotted, a complex attack is mounted. The immune system is spread throughout the body and involves many types of cells, organs, proteins, and tissues. Crucially, it can distinguish our tissue from foreign tissue — self from non-self. Dead and faulty cells are also recognized and cleared away by the immune system.[7]

Phase Six: Autonomic Nervous System

Phase six, is your autonomic nervous system (ANS). The ANS

includes two neurological constructs. The first is the sympathetic nervous system. The second is your parasympathetic nervous system.

The sympathetic side is known as your "fight or flight" aspect of your neurology. This system is triggered when we are in danger, surprised, scared, threatened, etc. Here is a quick example. Imagine you are driving down a quiet, tree-lined street. You have your favorite music on, there is a slight breeze in the air, the sun is shining… a perfect day. All of a sudden, you see a soccer ball bouncing into the street right toward your vehicle. Immediately after the ball, you now visualize a little boy quickly running after his ball. The problem in this story is that the boy is not paying attention to you or your car.

You literally have milliseconds to react to this stimulus. Thankfully, without really having to think about it, your nervous system kicks into hyperdrive. Your physiology responds in a very specific and dramatically rapid way. Your eyes are witnessing this event. Your eyes communicate with your brain. Your brain then signals the release of numerous chemicals and hormones such as adrenaline to be dumped into your bloodstream. Your acute awareness of this situation is now dialed in. The precision of events taking place so succinctly and efficiently inside of your body is magical. You barely have to think to slam on the brakes. You just do it. Crisis averted. The little boy is saved from massive injury because your finely-tuned sympathetic reflexes were triggered and acted upon. The sympathetic system engaged and you effectively responded. Success. The beautiful truth is you have moments like this multiple times per day, week, etc.

But, what if you are locked into a long-standing sensation of fear, pressure, mental tension? Granted it is not every day that you a thwarting dangerous soccer ball scenarios, but what if you sustained constant emotional stress? The kind of emotional stress that creates continual firing of your sympathetic nervous system. Think of the phrase "burning the candle from both ends".

Most people are not thinking about the impact everyday stress has on their health. Finances, relationships, career stresses left unchecked lead to ill-health because they tax and drain the sympathetic nervous system. This system runs on nutrition, too. In fact, your sympathetic nervous system runs on alkaline minerals such as magnesium, potassium, and sodium. Under extreme cases of sustained sympathetic stress, you lose vital alkaline balance within the body. This leads to acidity, pain, constipation, etc. Once again, you can pick a symptom and it can likely be traced back to some nutritional deficit such as the sympathetic nervous system being overworked. Every single day, we have tension in our lives. We're thinking about finances, and we're worried. We're thinking about our relationships and we're concerned. We're thinking about our kids and we're nervous. If these stresses are not reconciled, the system spins out of control and the body can no longer manage to remain in homeostasis. Remember, as we discussed in chapter 3, there are 3 forms of stress. They are emotional, nutritional, and physical in origin.

When you think in a stressful way, when you are stuck in that fight or flight response, you are losing your alkalinity, meaning, you're becoming acidic. Cancer thrives in an acid environment. If you are in this constant state of stress, you are potentially dumping potassium, magnesium, and sodium from your body.

Speaking of cancer, I felt this would be interesting to include. "The nature of cancer was first elucidated in 1902 by Scottish embryologist John Beard, PhD." 17,000 peer-reviewed papers about cancer research were found to be compatible with Beard's theory of the nature of cancer. Cancer cells from every tumor have the following in common:

- Low voltage +30 millivolts and the polarity is reversed in cancer cells (acidic pH)
- Lactic acid and sugar content are highly uniform
- Glucose can enter cancer cells but calcium and oxygen cannot
- Metabolism in cancer cells is anaerobic (lacking in oxygen)
- The concentration of eight B vitamins is nearly the same in all cancers
- The respiratory mechanism is essentially the same in all cancers
- The cytochrome oxidase content in cancers is essentially the same
- Liver catalase is depressed in all cancers
- All cancers have a uniformly low content of aerobic catalytic systems such as cytochrome, succinic, and d-amino acid oxidases, cytochrome-c, catalase and flavin.
- Cancers have elevated water and cholesterol content
- Induction of cancer by a single carcinogen causes cancers as diverse as leukemia and melanoma.
- Cancers have the ability to metastasize.[8] *Healing Is Voltage*

The second system within the ANS, is the parasympathetic nervous system. This system is known as the "feed and breed" system. This is the feel good aspect of your nervous system. The side of the nervous system highly in charge of digesting food and the pleasurable components to sexual activity. The parasympathetic nervous system runs on acidic minerals. Please understand that you need acidic minerals. These minerals include phosphorus, chloride, and sulfur. If you are under significant parasympathetic stress or dominance, one symptom you may encounter is anxiety. My experience is that it is very rare for someone to be significantly stressed in the parasympathetic nervous system. Without question, most people struggle with sympathetic dominance. More people are overly acidic versus being overly alkaline.

Phase Seven: The Endocrine System

Now, we're on to our seventh phase of digestive stress, which is the endocrine system. This is your hormone system. Because fats and proteins make your hormones, it is vital that you're eating enough of these key hormone-creating nutrients. Examples of high quality fats and proteins are going to be pastured eggs, wild-caught fish, organic meats, lentils, beans, avocados, avocado oil, coconuts, unrefined coconut oil, grass-fed butter, organic and high fat cheeses, macadamia nuts, walnuts, cashews, etc. Please note, you should be cooking with unrefined coconut oil, avocado oil, grass-fed butter, or ghee.

Do not cook with olive oil. When you heat olive oil it degrades the oil. It turns rancid and it is not a good product to consume. Use extra virgin olive oil for cold preparations for homemade salad dressings and dips.

Next, you should be eating *at least* 60 grams of fat and protein each day. Understand that protein is your healing nutrient. Protein is the only macronutrient responsible for energy, growth and repair, *and* homeostasis. Most people miss the mark and do not eat anywhere near enough of this essential macronutrient. They're coming in at 30 grams a day when I recommend at least 60 grams per day or more.

Essential compounds such as hemoglobin, insulin, thyroxine, serotonin, etc. are derived from the proteins in your diet. This is why I repeatedly state that protein is your healing nutrient. We need it. Please start consuming more protein. For the love of all things. Just listen to me on this. Your Endocrine system will thank you.

Side Note: If you are going to consume dairy products, I recommend high milk-fat dairy (2 or 4% fat content), and organic only. Limit your dairy. If I had a sixth belly buster, it would definitely be dairy.

Phase Eight: The Lymphatic System

We have finally made it to phase eight, which is your lymphatic system. Think of your lymphatics as your body's sewer system. When I test my patients, if signs of lymphatic stress are noted, I must start here. The process of reducing/removing the burden on the lymphatic system is paramount. As I have stated previously, the further down the stress cascade we go, the more problematic this person's digestive system is.

Pretend garbage pickup day in a big city stops. If garbage removal ends, that is not going to be a pretty scene, is it? Imagine the nasty effects uncollected garbage has on the surrounding neighborhoods. Now imagine if it is left for days, weeks, or even years. Consider what happens when your body is not properly removing its own garbage. Imagine the effect this toxic debris has on your tissues, organs, cells? Are you creating the mental picture? When your body ineffectively removes waste, where does it go? Really consider this. Where does it go? It accumulates. This then can lead to inflammation, low energy, irritability, constipation, Crohn's, painful joints, arthritis, and so on. The symptoms associated with a clogged waste removing system are endless. It is no shocker that one of my best selling products is called Smart Lymph because it's formulated to support a healthy lymphatic system. This is what protein enzymes do, they clean the blood, the garbage, etc. Proteases and the lymphatics are a match made in heaven.

Without question, we have covered a lot of material within the 8 phases of digestive stress. The question you may be asking now is… What can I do about it? How can I discover what phase of digestive stress I may be in?

Incorporating results-oriented protocols is what I am all about. Restoring your confidence in the body's ability to heal itself is my focus and that is where the GUT-Check Protocol comes in. I have a test you may want to consider. It is the testing method I have employed for over a decade. It is called the GUT-Check Protocol.

The GUT-Check Protocol is my proprietary system of analyzing what phase of digestive stress you are in. Quite simply, it is a leaky gut test. The difference is that instead of testing the blood for useless food allergies/sensitivities, I evaluate 14 specific digestive test points. Much of this information is derived via the urine. Urine shows the price your body is paying to stay in balance. The urine leaves many more digestive clues than blood, stool, or hair do. I like to call the blood the "spoiled brat of the body". I mean think of it, the blood really does get what it wants first. It is spoiled because this fluid is that important. Understand that it is typical for blood to come back normal in patients experiencing rheumatoid arthritis, gas, bloat, Crohn's, IBS, nausea, etc. This often leads to the medical doctor prescribing an anti-anxiety or anti-depressant to the patient because some MD's think the patient is literally making things up. These MD's make many of their patients feel small and belittled. So off they send them with a "it is all in your head" prescription pacifier.

> **"It is better to be hated for what you are than to be loved for what you are not."** - André Gide

In my office, I can easily say I work with the best patients around. I want you to know that it doesn't fall short on me when patients seek my care, that they do so with the risk of ridicule. Whether this comes from members of their family, their doctor, their friends, etc., I have tremendous respect for this healthy rebellion and going-against-the-grain posture. These are the outliers, and I want to specifically take this moment to say how much I value and enthusiastically applaud their courage.

The people I help, actually *want* help. They do not chase symptoms, instead they seek solutions. These are the brave people questioning the "authority" of traditional medicine. Making the decision to deviate from the broken medical model is rapidly catching on. I make it no secret that the broken medical model gets my vote for the Most Revolting Industry award. Far too many Americans still think throwing toxic poisons and pills at symptoms is the solution. Big Pharma's marketing messages have been wildly successful. In 2013, The Washington Post reported Americans spent a staggering $329.2 billion dollars on prescription medications! That tallies to about $1000 per American. There is work to do. My mission to save 5 million lives from the broken medical model is just.

Please pay attention to the Timeless Healing Principles as they will never change:

Principle #1 The body knows how to heal itself.

Principle #2: The body is constantly trying to stay in homeostasis.

Principle #3: The body's primary defense system, known as the immune system, lives in the gut.

We need to stop masking the symptoms of nutritional imbalances with prescription medications. Instead, we must opt for feeding the body what it *really* needs. Food. Please be mindful that Big Pharma's "promise" is usually not for your well-being but for their own profit.

The medical model is broken.

> **"All truth passes through three stages. First, it is ridiculed. Second, it is violently opposed. Third, it is accepted as being self-evident."**
> **- Arthur Schopenhauer, German philosopher**

I may be in the business of helping those with urgent and uncontrollable diarrhea, IBS, Crohn's and chronic constipation, but what I *really* do is help a grandmother have the confidence to get on an airplane so she may visit her grandkids again. I help the corporate executive conduct long meetings without worrying if his gut will behave. I help the mom of two complete 10K races without making extra bathroom pit-stops along the way.

Freedom.

Every example above is precisely about regaining *freedom.*

If you want to regain your freedom from the crappiest health conditions, you must abandon symptom chasing in favor of solution seeking. Food is the real medicine. Only nutrition will normalize function. Only nutrition supplies energy. Your level of energy is directly connected to how well you digest food. Prescription medications are not foods. Prescription medications do not supply energy to your body. In fact, they diminish and deplete energy stores. Prescription medications do not normalize function within the body. In fact, they disturb and disrupt human physiology.

Your digestive health can no longer be ignored. Inside your gut are all of the undeniable reasons for your current health. The solution to better health, energy and vitality is and always has been in your control. Your health is *your* responsibility.

Now, *right now*, is the time to refuse working with doctors who do not listen to you.
Now, *right now*, is the time to pay attention and work with your body's inner doctor.
Now, *right now*, is the time to embrace your body's elegant healing machinery.
Now, *right now*, is the time to focus on healing practices that actually support optimal function.

Now, *right now*, is time for your Gut Check. Will you listen?

References:

Chapter 2

1. Mendehlson, S., Robert. Confessions of a Medical Heretic. Contemporary Books; 1 edition p. 19. 1979.

2. Shinya, Hiromi. The Enzyme Factor. Council Oak Books. Introduction, p. 1. 2010.

3. Yance, R. Donald. Adaptogens In Medical Herbalism. Rochester, VT: Healing Arts Press.

4. Graphic: 2018 ranking of the global top 10 biotech and pharmaceutical companies based on net income (in billion U.S. dollars) Biotechs Graphic Accessed at: https://www.statista.com/statistics/272720/top-global-biotech-and-pharmaceutical-companies-based-on-net-income/

5. Graphic: The Washington Post. Swanson, Ana. Research v. Marketing Graphic. Accessed at: www.washingtonpost.com/news/wonk/wp/2015/02/11/big-pharmaceutical-companies-are-spending-far-more-on-marketing-than-research/?utm_term=.b0f29307b04f

6. New York Times. Article: Chon, Gina. Accessed at: www.nytimes.com/2016/09/02/business/dealbook/rising-drug-prices-put-big-pharmas-lobbying-to-the-test.html

7. National Health Expenditure Data. Accessed at: https://www.cms.gov/research-statistics-data-and-systems/statistics-trends-and-reports/nationalhealthexpenddata/nhe-fact-sheet.html 2016.

8. The Guardian. McGreal, Chris. How big pharma's money – and its politicians – feed the US opioid crisis. Accessed at: https://www.theguardian.com/us-news/2017/oct/19/big-pharma-money-lobbying-us-opioid-crisis 2017.

9. The Washington Post. Dennis, Brady. Journal of American Medical Association Study: Nearly 60 percent of Americans — the highest ever — are taking prescription drugs. Accessed at: https://www.washingtonpost.com/news/to-your-health/wp/2015/11/03/more-americans-than-ever-are-taking-prescription-drugs/?utmterm=.fc57dd0d6c60 2015.

10. Mercola, Joseph. Why are Americans Getting So Little in Return for the Highest Medical Bills on the Planet? Accessed at: https://articles.mercola.com/sites/articles/archive/2013/03/16/ high-health-care-costs.aspx 2013.

11. Hogshire, Jim. Pills-A-Go-Go: A Fiendish Investigation into Pill Marketing, Art, History & Consumption. Feral House; 1 edition Chapter 1, p. 5. 1999.

Chapter 3

1. Shinya, Hiromi. The Enzyme Factor. Council Oak Books. Introduction, p. 1. 2010.

2. Yance, R. Donald. Adaptogens In Medical Herbalism. Rochester, VT: Healing Arts Press. Chapter 2, p. 22. 2013.

3. Yance, R. Donald. Adaptogens In Medical Herbalism. Rochester, VT: Healing Arts Press. Chapter 2, p. 21. 2013.

4. Loomis, Howard. The Enzyme Advantage. 21st Century Nutri-

tion Publishing. Chapter 2, p. 46. 2015.

5. Yance, R. Donald. Adaptogens In Medical Herbalism. Rochester, VT: Healing Arts Press. Chapter 2, p. 21. 2013.

6. Article: Mercola, Joseph. Accessed at: https://articles.mercola.com/sites/articles/archive/2013/01/23/united-states-health-ranking.aspx

7. Loomis, Howard. The Enzyme Advantage. 21st Century Nutrition Publishing. Chapter 3, p. 65. 2015.

8. National Cancer Institute. Article: Psychological Stress and Cancer. Accessed at: https://www.cancer.gov/about-cancer/coping/feelings/stress-fact-sheet

9. Freedman, Joshua. The Physics of Emotion: Candace Pert on Feeling Good. Accessed at: https://www.6seconds.org/2007/01/26/the-physics-of-emotion-candace-pert-on-feeling-good 2007.

10. Yance, R. Donald. Adaptogens In Medical Herbalism. Rochester, VT: Healing Arts Press. Chapter 2, p. 20. 2013.

11. Loomis, Howard. The Enzyme Advantage. 21st Century Nutrition Publishing. Chapter 4, p. 101. 2015.

Chapter 5

1. Guthrie, A. Helen, and Picciano, Frances, Mary. Human Nutrition. Saint Louis, MO: Mosby. Chapter 1, p. 188. 1995.

2. Mahan, L. Kathleen, and Escott-Stump, Sylvia, Krause's Food, Nutrition, and Diet Therapy; Ninth Edition. Philadelphia, PA:

W.B. Saunders Company. p. 1. 1996.

3. Loomis, Howard. The Enzyme Advantage. 21st Century Nutrition Publishing. Chapter 3, p. 78. 2015.

4. Mahan, L. Kathleen, and Escott-Stump, Sylvia, Krause's Food, Nutrition, and Diet Therapy; Ninth Edition. Philadelphia, PA: W.B. Saunders Company. p. 4. 1996.

5. Guthrie, A. Helen, and Picciano, Frances, Mary. Human Nutrition. Saint Louis, MO: Mosby. Chapter 1, p. 2. 1995.

6. Guthrie, A. Helen, and Picciano, Frances, Mary. Human Nutrition. Saint Louis, MO: Mosby. Chapter 1, p. 2. 1995.

7. Loomis, Howard. The Enzyme Advantage. 21st Century Nutrition Publishing. Chapter 3, p. 92. 2015.

8. Mahan, L. Kathleen, and Escott-Stump, Sylvia, Krause's Food, Nutrition, and Diet Therapy; Ninth Edition. Philadelphia, PA: W.B. Saunders Company. p. 32. 1996.

9. Loomis, Howard. The Enzyme Advantage. 21st Century Nutrition Publishing. Chapter 3, p. 87. 2015.

10. Loomis, Howard. The Enzyme Advantage. 21st Century Nutrition Publishing. Chapter 3, p. 68. 2015.

11. Mahan, L. Kathleen, and Escott-Stump, Sylvia, Krause's Food, Nutrition, and Diet Therapy; Ninth Edition. Philadelphia, PA: W.B. Saunders Company. p. 17-18. 1996.

12. Mahan, L. Kathleen, and Escott-Stump, Sylvia, Krause's Food,

Nutrition, and Diet Therapy; Ninth Edition. Philadelphia, PA: W.B. Saunders Company. p. 66. 1996.

13. Shinya, Hiromi. The Enzyme Factor. Council Oak Books. Introduction, p. 2. 2010.

14. Tinker, Ben. Accessed at: https://www.cnn.com/2016/11/15/health/heartburn-medication-stroke-risk/index.html 2016.

15. Tinker, Ben. Accessed at: https://www.cnn.com/2016/11/15/health/heartburn-medication-stroke-risk/index.html 2016.

16. Tinker, Ben. Accessed at: https://www.cnn.com/2016/11/15/health/heartburn-medication-stroke-risk/index.html 2016.

17. Mahan, L. Kathleen, and Escott-Stump, Sylvia, Krause's Food, Nutrition, and Diet Therapy; Ninth Edition. Philadelphia, PA: W.B. Saunders Company. p. 63. 1996.

18. Tennant, Jerry. Healing Is Voltage Lexington, KY. p. 29. 2015.

19. Tennant, Jerry. Healing Is Voltage Lexington, KY. p. 28-29. 2015.

20. Loomis, Howard. The Enzyme Advantage. 21st Century Nutrition Publishing. Chapter 3, p. 96. 2015.

21. Yance, R. Donald. Adaptogens In Medical Herbalism. Rochester, VT: Healing Arts Press. Chapter 2, p. 21. 2013.

22. Mahan, L. Kathleen, and Escott-Stump, Sylvia, Krause's Food, Nutrition, and Diet Therapy; Ninth Edition. Philadelphia, PA: W.B. Saunders Company. p. 391. 1996.

23. Tennant, Jerry. Healing Is Voltage. Lexington, KY. p. 31. 2015.

Chapter 6

1. Shinya, Hiromi. The Enzyme Factor. Council Oak Books. Introduction, p. 2. 2010.

2. About Enzymes/Dr. Howell Accessed at: nationalenzyme.com/company-news/dr-edward-howellrevisited

3. About Enzymes/Dr. Howell Accessed at: www.enzyme-facts.com/dr-edward-howell.html

4. Howell, Edward. Enzyme Nutrition. Garden City, NY: Avery Publishing Group. Chapter 1, p. 1.1985.

5. About Enzymes/Dr. Howell. Accessed at: nationalenzyme.com/company-news/dr-edward- howellrevisited

6. About Enzymes/Dr. Howell. Accessed at: www.westonprice.org/health-topics/nutrition- greats/edward-howell-md

7. Loomis, Howard. The Enzyme Advantage. 21st Century Nutrition Publishing. Chapter 3, p. 71. 2015.

8. Howell, Edward. Enzyme Nutrition. Garden City, NY: Avery Publishing Group. Chapter 1, p. 3.1985.

9. Howell, Edward. Enzyme Nutrition. Garden City, NY: Avery Publishing Group. Chapter 1, p. 3.1985.

10. Howell, Edward. Enzyme Nutrition. Garden City, NY: Avery

Publishing Group. Chapter 2, p. 35.1985.

11. About Enzymes/Dr. Howell. Accessed at: www.westonprice. org/health-topics/nutrition- greats/edward-howell-md

12. Howell, Edward. Enzyme Nutrition. Garden City, NY: Avery Publishing Group. Chapter 2, p. 34-35.1985.

13. About Enzymes/Dr. Howell. Accessed at: www.westonprice. org/health-topics/nutrition- greats/edward-howell-md

14. Loomis, Howard. The Enzyme Advantage. 21st Century Nutrition Publishing. Chapter 3, p. 68. 2015.

15. Howell, Edward. Enzyme Nutrition. Garden City, NY: Avery Publishing Group. Chapter 2, p.xv-35.1985.

16. About Enzymes/Dr. Howell. Accessed at: www.westonprice. org/health-topics/nutrition- greats/edward-howell-md

17. About Enzymes/Dr. Howell. Accessed at: www.westonprice. org/health-topics/nutrition- greats/edward-howell-md

18. About Enzymes/Dr. Howell. Accessed at: www.westonprice. org/health-topics/nutrition- greats/edward-howell-md

19. About Enzymes/Dr. Howell. Accessed at: www.westonprice. org/health-topics/nutrition- greats/edward-howell-md

20. Howell, Edward. Enzyme Nutrition. Garden City, NY: Avery Publishing Group. Chapter 2, p. 41. 1985.

23. Tennant, Jerry. Healing Is Voltage. Lexington, KY. p. 31. 2015.

Chapter 6

1. Shinya, Hiromi. The Enzyme Factor. Council Oak Books. Introduction, p. 2. 2010.

2. About Enzymes/Dr. Howell Accessed at: nationalenzyme.com/company-news/dr-edward-howellrevisited

3. About Enzymes/Dr. Howell Accessed at: www.enzyme-facts.com/dr-edward-howell.html

4. Howell, Edward. Enzyme Nutrition. Garden City, NY: Avery Publishing Group. Chapter 1, p. 1. 1985.

5. About Enzymes/Dr. Howell. Accessed at: nationalenzyme.com/company-news/dr-edward-howellrevisited

6. About Enzymes/Dr. Howell. Accessed at: www.westonprice.org/health-topics/nutrition-greats/edward-howell-md

7. Loomis, Howard. The Enzyme Advantage. 21st Century Nutrition Publishing. Chapter 3, p. 71. 2015.

8. Howell, Edward. Enzyme Nutrition. Garden City, NY: Avery Publishing Group. Chapter 1, p. 3. 1985.

9. Howell, Edward. Enzyme Nutrition. Garden City, NY: Avery Publishing Group. Chapter 1, p. 3. 1985.

10. Howell, Edward. Enzyme Nutrition. Garden City, NY: Avery Publishing Group. Chapter 2, p. 35. 1985.

11. About Enzymes/Dr. Howell. Accessed at: www.westonprice. org/health-topics/nutrition-greats/edward-howell-md

12. Howell, Edward. Enzyme Nutrition. Garden City, NY: Avery Publishing Group. Chapter 2, p. 34-35. 1985.

13. About Enzymes/Dr. Howell. Accessed at: www.westonprice. org/health-topics/nutrition-greats/edward-howell-md

14. Loomis, Howard. The Enzyme Advantage. 21st Century Nutrition Publishing. Chapter 3, p. 68. 2015.

15. Howell, Edward. Enzyme Nutrition. Garden City, NY: Avery Publishing Group. Chapter 2, p. xv-35. 1985.

16. About Enzymes/Dr. Howell. Accessed at: www.westonprice. org/health-topics/nutrition-greats/edward-howell-md

17. About Enzymes/Dr. Howell. Accessed at: www.westonprice. org/health-topics/nutrition-greats/edward-howell-md

18. About Enzymes/Dr. Howell. Accessed at: www.westonprice. org/health-topics/nutrition-greats/edward-howell-md

19. About Enzymes/Dr. Howell. Accessed at: www.westonprice. org/health-topics/nutrition-greats/edward-howell-md

20. Howell, Edward. Enzyme Nutrition. Garden City, NY: Avery Publishing Group. Chapter 2, p. 41. 1985.

Chapter 7:

1. The Daily Mail. Prigg, Mark. How Animal Farm was right: Pigs really ARE almost identical to humans, say scientists. Accessed at: http://www.dailymail.co.uk/sciencetech/article-2232978/George Orwell-right-Pigs-really-ARE-identical-humans.html 2012.

2. Aflatoxins and Mold, and Cancer. Accessed at: https://www.cancer.gov/about-cancer/causes-prevention/risk/substances/aflatoxins

3. Genetically Modified Organisms. Accessed at: https://www.nongmoproject.org/

4. Philpott, Tom. GMO's and Indian Farmers: Accessed at: www.motherjones.com/food/2015/09/no-gmos-didnt-create-indias-farmer-suicide-problem/2015.

5. Shinya, Hiromi. The Enzyme Factor. Council Oak Books. Introduction, p. 91-92. 2010.

6. Bristol Stool Cart. Accessed at: https://www.webmd.com/digestive-disorders/poop-chart-bristol-stool-scale

7. Newman, Tim. How The Immune System Works. Accessed at: www.medicalnewstoday.com/articles/320101.php 2018.

8. Tennant, Jerry. Healing Is Voltage. Lexington, KY. p. 3. 2015.

Check out Dr. Christine's Podcast:

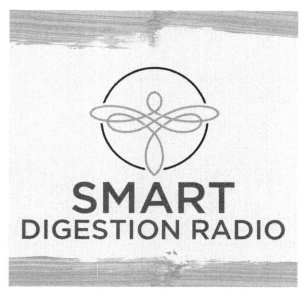

bit.ly/GutPodcast

To learn about Dr. Christine's
custom formulations:

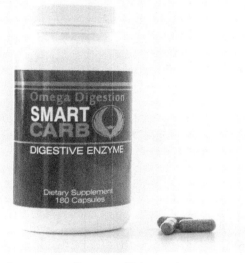

Visit www.OmegaDigestion.com

Notes:

Notes:

Notes:

Notes:

Notes:

Notes:

Notes:

Notes:

Made in United States
North Haven, CT
25 June 2023

38213805R00093